Eating Well for a Healthy Lifestyle

An Interesting Guide to Mind Your Eating Habits to Maintain a Perfect Balance in Life

By Anthony Elliott

Table of Contents

INTRODUCTION 1

CHAPTER 1: ABCS OF HEALTHY EATING 5

ANALYZE WHAT YOU EAT 5
BUILD HEALTHY EATING PRACTICES 19
    Making and Following a Diet Chart 19
    Checking One's Calorie Intake 20
    Reading Books About Eating Healthy 20
    Consulting a Dietitian 21
CONTROL YOUR EATING HABITS 21
    Aim for Eating Variety 22
    Make Healthy Choices of Food 22
    Eat Mindfully in Moderation 23

CHAPTER 2: COMPONENTS OF A HEALTHY EATING PLAN 25

DIETARY FIBER 27
    Best Fiber-Rich Diets 28
    Benefits of a High-Fiber Diet 28
WATER 29
    Food Rich in Water 30
    Benefits of Water in Diet 30
MACRO NUTRIENTS 31
    Carbohydrates 32
    Proteins 34
    Fats 36
MICRO NUTRIENTS 38
    Vitamins 38
    Minerals 42

CHAPTER 3: COUNT YOUR CALORIES 47

WHAT CALORIES ARE? 48
WHY COUNT YOUR CALORIES? 49
WHAT IS THE IDEAL CALORIE COUNT? 50
HOW TO COUNT YOUR CALORIE INTAKE? 51
ADVANCED CALORIE COUNTING APPS 59
BENEFITS TO COUNT YOUR CALORIES 61

CHAPTER 4: BEST DIET PLANS TO STAY HEALTHY 65

Low-Carb Diet 66
Ketogenic Diet 68
    Simple Diet Plans 71
    Health Benefits 71
Atkins Diet 72
    Sample Meal Plans 74
    Health Benefits 74
South Beach Diet 75
    Sample Meal Plans 77
    Health Benefits 77
Paleo Diet 78
    Sample Diet Plans 79
    Health Benefits 80
Dukan Diet 80
    Sample Meal Plans 82
    Health Benefits 82
Intermittent Diet 83
    Sample Diet Plans 85
    Health Benefits 85
Mediterranean Diet 86
    Sample Diet Plans 87
    Health Benefits 87
DASH Diet 88
    Sample Meal Plans 90
    Health Benefits 90
Vegan Diet 91
    Sample Meal Plan 93
    Health Benefits 93

CHAPTER 5: DOS AND DON'TS TO EAT WELL **95**

Dos For Healthy Eating 96
    Include Fruits and Vegetables in Your Diet 96
    Eat in Smaller Portions 97
    Stay Hydrated 97
    Follow a Diet Plan 98
    Track Your Meals 99
Don'ts For Healthy Eating 100
    Avoid Skipping Meals 100
    Limit Caffeine Intake 101
    Say No to Added Sugars 101
    Reduce Consumption of Junk Food 102
    Refrain from Alcohol 103

CHAPTER 6: PERKS OF HEALTHY EATING **105**

BOOSTS IMMUNITY 106

IMPROVES HEART HEALTH 107

STRENGTHENS TEETH AND BONES 107

MAINTAINS A HEALTHY BODY WEIGHT 108

ENHANCES DIGESTION 108

REDUCES STRESS 109

INCREASES LIFE EXPECTANCY 110

PROVIDES BETTER SLEEP 110

IMPROVES SKIN QUALITY 111

CHAPTER 7: OBSTACLES ON THE PATH OF EATING GOOD 113

LACK OF TIME TO PLAN EATING HABITS 114

EATING DISORDERS 115

Binge-Eating Disorder 115

Anorexia Nervosa 116

Bulimia Nervosa 116

Pica 117

Restrictive Food Intake Disorder 117

LACK OF KNOWLEDGE 118

CHAPTER 8: THREATS OF UNHEALTHY EATING HABITS 119

OBESITY 120

MALNUTRITION 121

Undernutrition 122

Overnutrition 122

HIGH CHOLESTEROL 123

FLUCTUATING BLOOD PRESSURE 124

VARIOUS DISEASES 125

DIGESTIVE ISSUES 125

Constipation 126

Gallstones 126

Diverticular Diseases 126

SLEEP DISORDERS 127

POOR EFFICIENCY 128

CHAPTER 9: MYTHS ABOUT HEALTHY EATING 129

EATING CARB-RICH FOOD IS UNHEALTHY 130

A VEGAN DIET IS A HEALTHIER OPTION 131

EATING FRUITS INCREASES BLOOD SUGAR 131

EATING FATTY FOODS WILL MAKE YOU FAT 132

CALORIES ARE ALWAYS UNHEALTHY 132

EAT BREAKFAST LIKE A KING 133

CHAPTER 10: GET INSPIRED TO EAT WELL 135

BRAD PITT 136

JENNIFER ANISTON 137

CHLOE BURROWS..137

LUCY LIU 138

TOM CRUISE 138

KATE HUDSON..139

CHAPTER 11: INTERESTING FACTS ABOUT HEALTHY EATING **141**

CONCLUSION..**149**

REFERENCES **151**

IMAGE REFERENCES 160

Introduction

Keeping your body healthy is an expression of gratitude to the whole cosmos—the trees, the clouds, everything. –Thich Nhat Hanh, a Vietnamese Monk

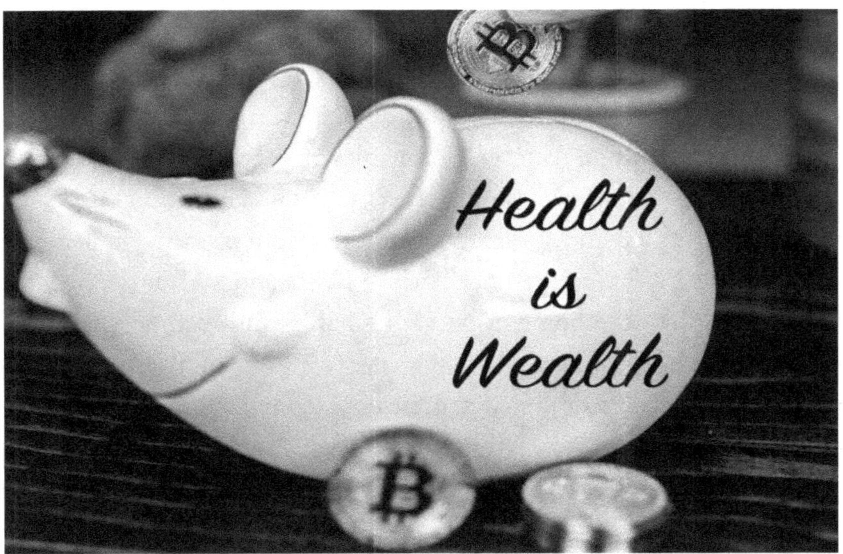

In today's high-tech and fully mechanized world, where we need to move at a very fast pace to match up with all the dynamic activities of our life, staying happy and healthy is a big challenge for all of us. Our life is a blessing, which can be visualized as the beautiful creation of our active lifestyle, optimistic thinking, and healthy eating habits. Apparently, in the race to accomplish our daily chores and to meet the increasing demands of livelihood, one easily gears up into an active mode of living. But, while doing so, we often overlook the fact that by adopting such an active lifestyle, we are putting ourselves at a higher risk of disturbing our mental peace and physical well-being. In this regard, Thich Nhat Hanh has strongly expressed his views in the above-mentioned quote, by highlighting the fact that we need to be thankful to the whole universe for helping us maintain our health, as everything around us contributes to the path of this arduous journey of staying fit and healthy. Thus, our health is not something that is just an internal factor alone, instead, it is governed by what our surrounding is like, how we maintain our lifestyle, what we eat to survive, and many more such interesting factors.

Pondering over the most important of all i.e., eating, which can be a passion, love, interest, some type of disorder, or simply a means of survival for many people. Today's, fashion and health-oriented society is pushing the crowd toward the race of looking good, gorgeous, and glamorous. But, during the course of achieving it, we often overlook the fact that just good looks and outer beauty won't last for long unless we have a healthy mind and soul. However, this chimera of life vanishes off sooner or later, as we encounter the truth of life and look at the healthier side of living by developing good eating habits and maintaining a well-balanced lifestyle. Expressing his views, Benjamin Franklin has beautifully emphasized the importance of eating in our lives, in his mesmerizing quote mentioned below:

Eat to live, don't live to eat, Benjamin Franklin, an American writer

The journey to eat healthily, begins from knowing about and exploring the hidden treasures of nature that we are blessed with, to eat and enjoy our living. If we spare some time and think wisely, we will realize that we have a wide range of diversity, when it comes to selecting what to eat. However, this selection is based on our personal choices, whether to opt for plant-based food items or animal-based food products is in our own hands. Apart from this, it is also necessary to develop good habits that promote and encourage healthy eating like making a daily diet chart, counting your calories, consulting a dietitian, following a good diet plan, and many more. But, for following all these things religiously and making them an intact part of our lives, we need to have the willpower and determination to make a change in our lifestyle. This is possible only when we have the power to control ourselves against indulgence in unhealthy eating habits, any sort of cravings for food, or adopting a sedentary and sluggish life pattern. So, we can consider healthy eating as a package, that demands both physical and mental coordination to work wonders for us in the journey of life.

Many of us love to explore and enjoy trying new varieties of food, but to our surprise, hardly a few of us may be interested to know what type of food we are eating, what quantity is sufficient for our body, what are the benefits of eating the food we consume, how that food works to keep us fit and healthy in a long run, and many such engaging questions. Thus, by diving deeper into the science of eating healthy, we can learn about the different important components of food i.e., fats, carbohydrates, proteins, vitamins, and minerals. Along with that, it is also necessary to track the amount of calories that we are consuming in each of our meals, in a day. With technological developments, lack of time cannot be an excuse to keep oneself updated with the basics of one's diet, as there are various diet regulating and calorie tracking apps, that are just a touch away. Once we are all set for our journey to attain good eating habits, we are halfway done, but we cannot overlook the fact that the road toward goodness is often filled with thorns and spikes, as there can be many possible challenges and problems on our way to achieving sound health by inculcating good eating habits in ourselves.

In the journey of this whole process, we confront various benefits that we can earn from developing good and healthy eating habits, which can thereby help us stand strong against different obstacles and threats that may become a part and parcel of this alluring expedition. While we pass through the myriad phases of adopting eating as our healthy habit, it is we who will have to differentiate between a series of facts and myths that may make the process more challenging by creating delusions and doubts about what we are doing. But, as we look around us, we will surely realize that the race for staying fit by eating healthy has already begun and we have numerous shining and inspirational faces that set live examples for us, to achieve our goal with excellence and follow a healthy pattern of eating. Hence, the wait is over and the time has come to think twice before you eat! At this point in time, there may be various questions that may be hovering in your mind and creating unrest, as it is a bit difficult to get started with any new good habit. So, close your eyes, take a deep breath, visualize yourself as a fitness freak, and just follow the footsteps guided by us to unveil each and every step toward achieving good eating habits.

Chapter 1:

ABCs of Healthy Eating

Healthy eating is a way of life, so it's important to establish routines that are simple, realistically, and ultimately livable. —Horace, a Roman Poet

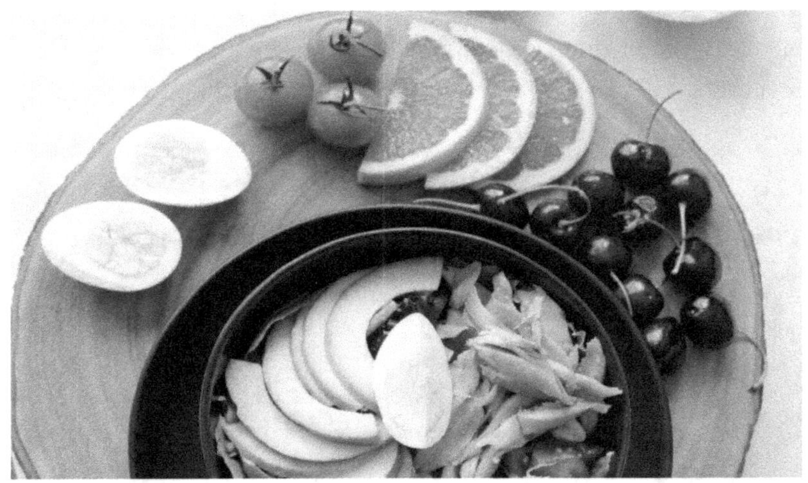

Eating healthy is not a complicated science that needs to be studied or researched, instead, this process of exploring the different types of food items and their vital elements can be made a fun-filled process by putting in some effort in the right direction. So, here we have simplified the whole process of healthy eating for you, by defining its ABCs in depth.

Analyze What you Eat

Eating is something that almost all living beings enjoy, but not all of us are mindful about what we are eating and while doing so we tend to consume whatever comes before us. In today's world, there are so many alluring and mouth-watering delicacies that may compel us to develop a craving or liking for them, eventually, making us feast on all the healthy and unhealthy choices. However, we get many different alternatives at every step of our life, but making a perfect and healthy choice is always in our own hands. When we talk about eating, it is we who will decide whether to have a fatty cheesy burger or a bowl of healthy green salad for our meal. The choice is all ours! But the biggest question arises on how to decide what is good and healthy for us in terms of eating, as many of us don't even know the basic components of food and the benefits of eating each one of them. There are a large variety of food products that are available to us in different forms and are obtained from different sources:

Sources		Examples	Benefits
Plants	Fruits	<ul><li>Apple</li><li>Blackberries</li><li>Pear</li><li>Raspberries</li></ul>	<ul><li>These fruits are rich in dietary fiber.</li><li>They aid in proper bowel movement.</li><li>They also assist in reducing the cholesterol levels in our body.</li></ul>
		<ul><li>Strawberries</li><li>Oranges</li><li>Red Peppers</li></ul>	<ul><li>These fruits are rich in vitamin C.</li><li>They help to boost the immune system.</li><li>They aid in maintaining strong teeth and healthy gums.</li></ul>

	• Mangoes • Bananas • Guavas • Cantaloupe	• These fruits have a high content of potassium. • They assist in maintaining a proper fluid balance in our body. • They also regulate blood pressure.
	• Prunes • Black Plums • Berries	• These fruits are a rich source of antioxidants. • They help in providing healthy and glowing skin. • They protect our bodies from various illnesses.
Vegetables	• Potato • Corn • Kale	• Eating Vegetables contribute to dietary fibers in our diet, which improves digestion. • These veggies are a great source of carbohydrates which are helpful in gaining weight at a faster rate.

• Cauliflower • Broccoli • Spinach • Beetroot • Carrots	• These green leafy vegetables when consumed regularly, help in shedding weight. • These vegetables are rich in potassium which helps regulate normal blood pressure. • They work wonders by reducing the chance of kidney stone formation. • They have loads of vitamin A and help in maintaining good eyesight. •
• Tomatoes • Lemon	• These citrus vegetables are a good source of vitamin C and help boost immunity. • They also help to maintain good skin health.

| Cereals | <ul><li>Wheat</li><li>Lentils</li><li>Barley</li><li>Rice</li></ul> | <ul><li>These cereals are a good source of cholesterol-free, fiber-rich diet.</li><li>They have a high content of phytochemicals and antioxidants, that lowers blood cholesterol.</li><li>They also contain a variety of vitamins and minerals, hence boosting immunity.</li><li>The high content of fiber in these cereals makes them helpful in improving digestion by adding on to roughage.</li></ul> |

Legumes	<ul><li>Kidney Beans</li><li>Black Beans</li><li>Green Peas</li><li>Chickpeas</li></ul>	<ul><li>Almost all the beans are low in fat content.</li><li>These legumes are a rich source of fiber, protein, vitamin B, and many vital minerals like zinc, potassium, phosphorous, etc.</li><li>For a vegan diet, one can easily replace the protein obtained from meat and dairy products with that in lentils.</li><li>These legumes contain antioxidants that help our body to efficiently fight against diseases and delay aging.</li></ul>

Spices	<ul><li>Cinnamon</li><li>Sage</li><li>Turmeric</li><li>Rosemary</li><li>Cardamom</li><li>Cumin Seeds</li><li>Carom Seeds</li></ul>	<ul><li>Cinnamon helps in lowering blood sugar and works wonders for those suffering from diabetes.</li><li>Sage is a miracle spice, as it helps to improve brain functioning, boosts memory, and also fights against Alzheimer's disease.</li><li>Turmeric exhibits anti-inflammatory action and aids in the quick healing of wounds.</li><li>Rosemary is well-known for its benefits in fighting allergic responses and nasal congestion.</li><li>Cardamom helps suppress the feeling of nausea and is a great flavoring agent in various food items.</li></ul>

Beverages	<ul><li>Green Tea</li><li>Herbal Tea</li><li>Milk Tea</li><li>Milk Coffee</li><li>Black Coffee</li></ul>	<ul><li>Tea and coffee have certain chemicals within them called antioxidants, that help to fight the free radicals which have the tendency to damage our body cells and cause various illnesses.</li><li>Caffeine present in tea and coffee, helps in providing protection against Parkinson's disease.</li><li>Green tea works wonders in shedding weight.</li><li>Herbal tea has the benefits of many herbs in it, which help our body fight various health problems like constipation, sleep disorders, common cold, etc.</li></ul>

Oils	<ul><li>Coconut Oil</li><li>Sunflower Oil</li><li>Olive Oil</li><li>Soya Bean Oil</li><li>Flaxseed Oil</li></ul>	<ul><li>These plant-based oils are rich in omega-3 fatty acids that are healthy for our body.</li><li>These oils are trans-fat free and hence help to lower blood cholesterol.</li><li>They also maintain normal blood pressure and hence reduce the risk of coronary heart diseases, strokes, type-2 diabetes, and heart attacks.</li><li>These plant-based oils are a great source of fat-soluble vitamins i.e Vitamin A, D, E, and K.</li></ul>

| Non-Dairy Milk | • Almond Milk
• Soy Milk
• Oat Milk
• Cashew Milk | • Almond milk is the best source of non-dairy milk, as it is low on calories, is less fatty, and has zero cholesterol.
• Soy milk, when compared to other non-dairy milk has the highest protein content.
• Oat milk has soluble fibers that dissolve in water and form a gel-like substance in our stomach while digestion, thereby slowing down the process and making us feel full for a longer time.
• Cashew milk has anti-cancer properties due to the antioxidants present in it. |

| Animals | Milk | <ul><li>Cow's Milk</li><li>Goat's Milk</li><li>Buffalo Milk</li></ul> | <ul><li>Milk can be consumed in a variety of forms like cheese, butter, yogurt, cream, etc.</li><li>It is considered to be a complete food, as it contains almost all the vitamins and minerals that are required for the proper growth and development of mind and body.</li><li>Milk is the best source of good fats, high-quality proteins, and carbs in the form of lactose.</li><li>It is rich in calcium and thus helps in maintaining healthy teeth and bones.</li></ul> |

Meat		• White Meat • Red Meat	• All bird meat like chicken, turkey, quail, goose, etc., fall under the category of white meat. • Meat is also available in processed forms like hotdogs, sausages, luncheons, bacon, etc. • Red Meat is rich in a protein called myoglobin that has high iron content and is helpful in making one active by providing extra oxygen. • Experts suggest consuming white meat over red meat due to cancer risks that are associated with red meat.
Eggs		• Chicken Eggs • Quail Eggs • Duck Eggs • Turkey Eggs	• Eggs are a major source of protein in our diet. • It increases good cholesterol and hence reduces the risk of stroke and various heart diseases. • It is rich in vitamin A which helps to maintain good eyesight.

Seafood	Freshwater Fish	<ul><li>Catfish</li><li>Trout</li><li>Bass</li><li>Whitefish</li></ul>	<ul><li>It is the best choice for a high-protein, low-fat diet.</li><li>They are packed with many vitamins and minerals that help to maintain healthy hair and skin.</li></ul>
	Salt Water Fish	<ul><li>Salmon</li><li>Tuna</li><li>Halibut</li><li>Cod</li></ul>	<ul><li>They are a great source of omega-3 fatty acids as compared to the other freshwater fishes, thereby enhancing the functioning of the heart.</li><li>They are low in mercury content and are thus more preferred over freshwater fishes.</li></ul>

Shellfish	• Crabs • Shrimps • Lobsters • Scallops • Oysters	• It is a healthy choice for those looking for an alternative to meat. • They are rich in minerals like selenium and zinc, which are vital for the proper functioning of our body. • They are an abundant source of protein and have less fat content which makes them a favorite of seafood lovers. • They can be cooked in various ways like steamed, baked, or grilled to enhance their taste.
Roe Caviar	• Eggs of Fish	• They are a good source of proteins and can be used fresh or can also be canned to use later. • Caviar is a high-end product of fish belonging to the sturgeon family and is expensive as compared to roe.

Build Healthy Eating Practices

To select the best meal plan for oneself, one needs to be aware of what are the different available options that can be healthy and beneficial for our body. In simple words, we can elaborate that healthy eating includes all the food items that help us stay mentally alert and physically active. It is necessary to maintain a perfect balance between the different elements of food that will be discussed in detail in the coming chapters, to create a clear picture of what to eat and what to leave. Apart from this, one needs to organize their eating habits by inculcating a few good and healthy practices, like:

Making and Following a Diet Chart

Many of us may find it a challenging task, to follow a fixed diet plan or eat according to the diet prescribed by the dietitian. So, all those looking out for some flexibility in their eating patterns, budget, and taste; can surely go ahead with making their own diet chart. This can be very helpful as one can decide accordingly, what to eat and in what quantity, in order to meet the daily requirements of all the essential nutrients. The most important thing that matters while making a diet chart is your goal or motive, as it helps you to easily sort out the best and most feasible food items, in terms of their calorie count and nutrient content. Once a diet chart is prepared, you need to follow it regularly to see the desired changes in your lifestyle. So, with your strong willpower and self-determination, you can really make a difference in your life, in your own style.

Checking One's Calorie Intake

Eating food without being conscious of its calorie content can prove to be a disaster for those who aim to stay healthy and fit, as it leads to an uncontrolled intake of food items. Every food item has its own calorie count, which needs to be tracked or explored before consuming any food or even while making a diet chart of your own. Counting calories is one of the healthiest eating habits that one can inculcate in their life easily, as with the advancement in technology, exploring anything is just a touch away. Nowadays, with the help of a number of apps and web pages, you can extract the data for the calorie count of various food items with ease. Moreover, there are many calorie-counting apps, that can assist you in counting your calories, effortlessly. So, eating in a healthy and balanced way can surely help one manage their weight and maintain the overall health of the body.

Reading Books About Eating Healthy

If you are a foodie, then one of the best ways to keep yourself updated with interesting food facts and pieces of information is by reading books about healthy eating. Sitting peacefully with a cup of hot coffee and exploring many new things about a variety of food items and eating habits, is something very soothing and comforting. Nowadays, you can opt for e-books or audiobooks too, in order to enjoy a hassle-free time reading and enjoying the content of the book. There are loads of diverse and unexplored things, that each book conveys in its own style. So, just go for the right book according to your taste and dive deep into the ocean of words, that will indeed take you away to another mesmerizing world of delicious delicacies.

Consulting a Dietitian

In life, there are times when after trying many different diet plans and making your own diet charts, you still feel confused and unsatisfied with your health progress as you don't see the desired results. Then, it's time to approach the dietitian and seek some good pieces of advice about maintaining proper and healthy eating habits. A dietitian will first monitor your weight and examine you for your physical fitness, then he will talk to you about your goals and targets that you would like to achieve in a particular time span. After enquiring about the basic details of your health, the dietitian will recommend you some courses that have been planned especially for you, in order to get closer to your targeted health goals. The dietitian will stay in touch will you, to track your health progress and guide you with the dos and don'ts during the course. So, consulting a dietitian will actually reduce your burden of carving the pathway to attain good health.

Control Your Eating Habits

One of the biggest challenges in the endeavor to achieve healthy eating, is to develop the willpower and courage to control oneself against the cravings and desires to eat whatever is before us, without reckoning what it may bring to us in return. There are many people among us who tend to overeat in a sitting by consuming too many calories in a go, or simply eat because they are bored or tense exhibiting signs of stress eating disorder. Thus, many times we don't eat consciously, instead, we fail to control our instinct of eating. We can try to get out of this mess, by diverting our minds away from eating or by meditating to increase our willpower and focus. Studies have revealed that by doing so, we can move one step ahead toward controlling our urge to munch. However, this process is a time taking one, but we can keep our morale high by adding some fun-filled activities for ourselves like fasting for a few hours a week, cutting down a few of our favorite unhealthy snacks, taking up the challenge of eating fruits only, and many such creative ideas.

Aim for Eating Variety

Many of us often love to munch on our favorite food items thereby overlooking the concept behind a balanced diet. However, experts around the world, emphasize including a variety of different food items in our daily diet plan, which will eventually boost our overall body metabolism and help to fight against various chronic diseases. Moreover, following a well-balanced diet that contains all the vital components of food in the required ratios, will also be beneficial to combat the raising issues of malnutrition and obesity. Thus, when we talk of healthy eating, it's not just the quantity or the quality of food that is to be considered, instead, it refers to good quality food that is taken in the right amount and right proportion, that can really make a visible change in our lifestyle.

Make Healthy Choices of Food

Life always allures us by presenting many tempting options before us, but making a choice that is perfect and healthy is always in our hands. The same thing applies when it comes to choosing our daily meals. Thus, whether to opt for a bowl of fruits or a big slice of cheesy pizza, completely depends on our willpower and intention. So, whenever you get an opportunity to go ahead with making a decision about what to eat, you should always choose wisely by keeping in mind the calorie requirements of your body and the nutritional value of different food items in your diet chart. This will surely form a strong base, for moving ahead with a healthier eating option in life.

Eat Mindfully in Moderation

At times, we get carried away by the temptations of our favorite food and don't even realize that we are indulging in the harmful act of overeating. In simple words, munching on our most loved food item is termed as overeating and it is the root cause of many serious health issues like obesity, high cholesterol, chronic heart disorders, etc. On the contrary, when preoccupied with all the worldly tensions and worries, we often fail to focus on eating properly, which may result in a lack of nutrition that is necessary for staying fit and healthy. Thus, mindfully eating our food will create conscious eating habits and help us to make a perfect balance in our life.

Chapter 2

Components of a Healthy Eating Plan

Healthy eating isn't about counting fat grams, dieting, cleanses and antioxidants; it's about eating food untouched from the way we find it in nature in a balanced way. –Pooja Mottl, an Author

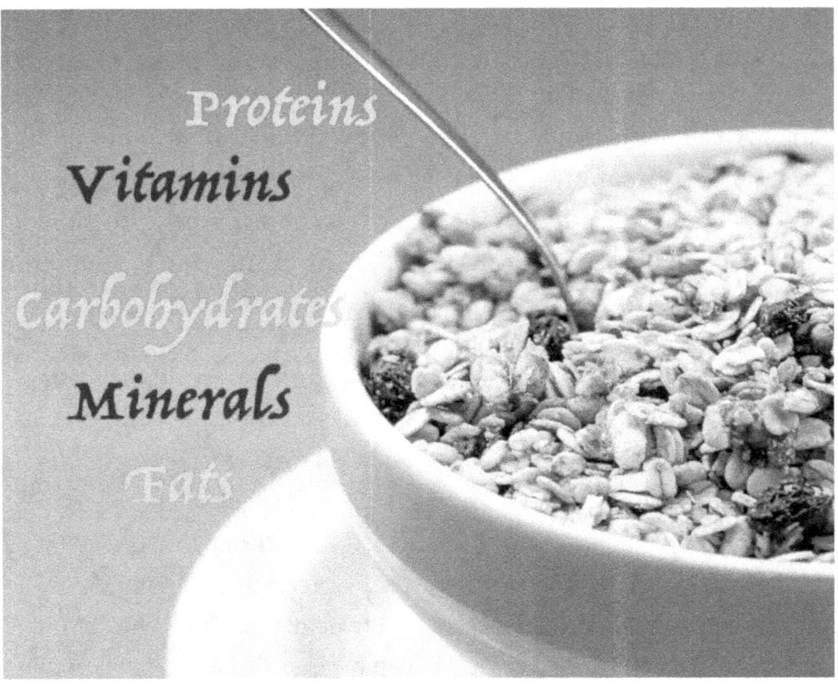

Achieving a balanced and healthy lifestyle, demands cumulative efforts in the field of understanding and learning the basics of eating a good diet. Thus, to develop and maintain our physical health, we need to work

toward reducing illness and boosting our mental well-being. Often, busy in the hustle and bustle of our lives we tend to ignore the needs of our body and don't bother to care for ourselves, which ultimately degrades our physical health and also affects our psychological presence. Despite being updated in this hi-tech world, many of us are still unaware of the secrets that can lead us toward maintaining a good and healthy lifestyle. One of the key factors that impact our health is the type of eating habits that we follow. If consumed in a balanced way, the food we eat can prove to be the best source of nutrition for us and improve our overall health. On the contrary, indulging in bad eating habits can become the prime reason behind several types of chronic diseases and health problems in our life. In simple words, the food we eat will probably decide, which health issues and diseases we are inviting toward us and at what pace. Apart from this, eating habits are also responsible for showing up the symptoms of aging in our body, thereby impacting our life expectancy too. However, developing a healthy lifestyle is not an overnight game-changing plan. Instead, it is a slow journey of building strong willpower, putting in consistent efforts, and gaining knowledge about the several aspects of eating healthy food. This can eventually help in providing complete nourishment to our body, by fulfilling the daily nutrient requirements in the best possible way.

Emerging technologies in this dynamically growing world, have created a great shift in our living styles, which has also influenced our eating habits drastically. Nowadays, food items that have a higher content of unhealthy fats, sodium, and sugar are easily available and seem to be more appealing to our taste buds than the healthier ones, resulting in enough damage to our health and fitness. Consuming such kinds of food regularly and for longer periods, gradually begins to show the symptoms and increases the risk of various chronic heart diseases, cardiovascular diseases, and other health problems like diabetes and obesity. These are the most common health issues that have set their strong foot not only into the lives of adults and older people but also affect the health of teenagers and younger kids. The root cause of these disturbed eating habits is the lack of awareness about the food that is crucial to maintain a healthy lifestyle and could help in achieving balanced and complete nutrition. So, let's delve into and understand the important components of food which are essential for achieving a balanced and nutritious diet to maintain a healthy lifestyle.

Dietary Fiber

Dietary Fiber, commonly called bulk or roughage, is that part of the plant that cannot be digested by our body. Unlike the other nutrients which are consumed and absorbed in the body, dietary fiber is not digested. Rather, these fibers move through the stomach to the small intestine, and colon and then gradually excreted out from the body. Dietary fibers form an important part of consuming a healthy and balanced diet as it severs numerous health benefits. Based on the solubility in water, dietary fibers are classified as:

1. Soluble Fibers: The soluble fiber can be easily dissolved into water and gastrointestinal fluids when it enters the stomach or intestines. It forms a gel-like substance, which is further digested in the large intestines or colon which releases calories and gases.

2. Insoluble Fibers: The insoluble dietary fibers are unable to get dissolved when they enter the intestines or stomach and are left unchanged while moving through the digestive tract. As these fibers cannot be digested at all, they are not a source of calories. Rather, insoluble fibers are essential for maintaining and promoting the movement of digested material throughout the digestive system. This is beneficial for increasing the stool bulk and helps in solving the problems of those who face issues of irregular stools or constipation.

Best Fiber-Rich Diets

A healthy diet is comprised of both types of dietary fiber be it soluble or insoluble fiber, because of the health benefits. The amount of soluble and insoluble fibers found in several plant-based sources vary from each other. To extract maximum benefits from dietary fibers, one must try to consume a balanced diet that is comprised of higher-fiber foods. The most common sources of soluble fiber are citric fruits and carrots. Beans, barley, oats, peas, apples, and psyllium. While, the rich sources of insoluble fibers are beans, nuts, wheat bran, whole-wheat flour, and several vegetables like potatoes, cauliflower, and green beans.

Benefits of a High-Fiber Diet

1. Normalizing the Bowel Movement: A diet that is rich in fiber helps in increasing the size and weight of the stool and helps in softening it. This makes it easy for the intestines to pass the bulk stool than compared to the loose and watery stools, which helps in easing and solving the issue of constipation. Dietary fibers help in absorbing the water from loose and watery stools and solidifying them.

2. Improving Bowel Health: A fiber-rich diet is also known for its benefits of reducing the risk of several diseases like colorectal cancer, hemorrhoids, and diverticular diseases. Diverticular disease is an inflammatory condition of the colon that mostly occurs in older adults. However, consuming a fiber-rich diet helps in cutting the risk of this disease by 40%.

3. Lowering cholesterol Level: Flaxseeds, oats, beans, and oat brans are rich in soluble fiber that reduces the low-density lipoprotein level, which helps in maintaining a suitable cholesterol level. Soluble fiber prevents the breakdown and digestion of dietary

cholesterol which gradually helps in reducing the cholesterol level in the blood.

4. Stabilizing blood glucose level: Soluble fiber prevents the digestion of several nutrients including carbohydrates. This helps in reducing the absorption rate of sugar in the blood, which stabilizes blood glucose levels. Thus, consuming a meal that is rich in soluble fiber could prevent sharp increases in blood sugar.

5. Maintaining a healthy weight: Consuming a high-fiber diet can help in feeling fuller for longer periods which reduces the need for eating at irregular intervals and unhealthy snacking. Further, fiber-rich food has low energy density, providing fewer calories as compared to other food, which can help in achieving a healthy weight.

Water

Water constitutes about two-thirds of our entire body weight and is essential for performing several important functions. Water supports the cells, tissues, and organs to perform their core functions and also regulate an optimum temperature. It helps in maintaining the fluid level of blood vessels to ensure a smooth and regular flow of blood in the stream. It also supports the body in eliminating the by-products of metabolism, excessive electrolytes like potassium and sodium, and urea. Apart from this, several other important functions of water are to assist in digestion, prevent constipation, nourish the skin, regulate body temperature through sweating, and carry oxygen and nutrients to the cells.

We can survive without solid food for weeks, however, without water, it can last only for a few days. Therefore, it is necessary to drink enough water that can support the body to function properly and efficiently. The amount of fluid required by our body depends upon various vital factors like age, gender, activity, lifestyle, and pregnancy or breastfeeding. People living in cold weather conditions, consuming a lot of fluid-rich food, or having a sedentary lifestyle may require less water. However, those who are following a high-fiber diet, and high-protein diet, live in warm weather conditions, do vigorous exercises, have an active lifestyle, or suffer from diarrhea or vomiting must consume higher amounts of water.

Food Rich in Water

Water can be derived from solid as well as liquid food sources. Almost all food items contain water, even if it is dry and hard. Solid food is enough to fulfill at least 20% of the daily water requirement in our body. The metabolism process during digestion also produces a small amount of water, as its by-product. This helps to provide at least 10% of the total water requirement by the body. While, the leftover 70% of the water requirement in the body must be obtained from various liquid sources like juice, healthy drinks and beverages, and water itself.

Benefits of Water in Diet

1. Creates Saliva: Saliva, a liquid that is produced by the salivary glands is made of electrolytes, enzymes, and mucus with its main component being water. Saliva is an important fluid that is secreted in the mouth and helps in breaking down several solid foods. A higher intake of water helps in producing more saliva which is good for keeping the mouth healthy.

2. Protect Body Organs: Water is vital for keeping the joints, spinal cord, and tissues healthy. Water works like a lubricant and provides a cushioning effect to the joints, tissues, and spinal

cords that supports performing several physical activities easily without any discomfort.

3. Removes Waste from the Body: An adequate amount of water intake supports the body in getting rid of several wastes and by-products through sweating, urination, and bowel movement. Sweating helps in regulating the temperature of the body and also removes the excess impurity from the skin. Drinking a good amount of water can help in supplementing the lost water through sweat. Apart from this, water is also required for avoiding constipation and having a healthy stool. Further, adequate water intake keeps the kidney health, as it uses water to purify the blood and filter out waste. Ensuing an optimum intake of water can help in avoiding kidney stones.

4. Supports Digestion and Nutrient Absorption: Drinking a good amount of water before a meal and during the meal is one of the best ways to support an easy breakdown of food and improve digestion. Apart from this, water also eases the absorption of several important vitamins, minerals, and nutrients from food and delivers them to the other parts of the body.

Macro Nutrients

As the name suggests, macronutrients are the major nutrients that are needed by our body in large quantities. Macronutrients help in generating energy and calories for maintaining the proper functioning of our body's systems and structure. These prime nutritive components include carbohydrates, fats, and protein which must not be manipulated in any form as they can have a serious impact on the proper functioning of the body. Many of the diets, plan to focus on changing and regulating the number of fats, proteins, and carbohydrates that must be consumed on an average daily. However, a healthy diet does not exclude or restrict the intake of any of these macronutrients.

Macronutrients cannot be produced inside our body on their own, instead, these nutrients are derived from several food items through an outside source. Choosing a healthy and balanced diet is one of the best ways to nourish our body with these macronutrients that form the basis of our inside functioning. However, having prior knowledge of the vital sources of macronutrients is important to opt for a healthy and balanced diet. A balanced diet is a core of developing a healthy lifestyle by focusing on a proportioned diet that stresses in consumption of every type of food item but in regulated and controlled amounts only.

Carbohydrates

Carbohydrates, often known as carbs or the primary fuel of our body, help in providing energy to the different muscles and nervous systems for doing vigorous exercises and movement throughout the entire day. On average, around 45 to 60% of the calories must be derived from the prime sources of carbohydrates, however, this can vary for each individual depending upon their medical and health condition. Our body breaks down carbohydrates into glucose that can easily circulate and be absorbed by every cell and tissue of our body. Carbohydrates are divided into simple and complex carbs based on their level of breakdown and absorption in our body. Simple carbs are made up of smaller chain molecules that can be easily absorbed and digested in our bodies. While complex carbs are the longer chains of molecules that take time to digest and stay longer in our blood in the form of glucose providing energy for doing daily activities and tasks. However, unhealthy food items like sweetened beverages and refined sugar are the most common source of simple carbs which makes it bad for our health. Therefore, it is recommended to opt for food items that are a good source of complex carbs and could help in providing energy to the body.

Food Rich in Carbohydrates

Carbohydrates can be derived from both healthy as well unhealthy sources, so it must be a wise decision to choose from the list. The most common healthy sources of carbs are the ones that are rich in vitamins, fiber, minerals, and phytochemicals. Phytochemicals are plant-based compounds that help the body to fight against several illnesses and diseases. The healthy sources of carbs are fresh vegetables, fruits, grains, and beans.

Apart from this, several sources of unhealthy carbohydrates are highly processed foods, soda, beverages, pastries, bread, and refined sugar. This food is easily digested and could also cause spikes in blood sugar which can increase the risk of several health conditions like obesity, diabetes, and heart diseases.

Benefits of Carbs in Diet

1. Provides Energy: Carbohydrates work like the fuelling agent in our body that provides the energy to stay active for the entire day. The food that is rich in carbs is digested in our body from sugar and starches to glucose which is easily absorbed into the bloodstream often called blood sugar. These carbs in the form of glucose are an active source of energy to do several tasks like jogging, workout or simply walking and thinking.

2. Protects Against Diseases: Food rich in carbohydrates are also a vital source of phytochemical, which are known for improving and boosting the immune system that automatically reduces the risk of diabetes, aging, inflammatory signs, and healing properties. Further, these are also famous for their antioxidant,

antidepressant, and wound-healing quality. Apart from this, phytochemical also helps in reducing the cancer cell growth rate and preventing DNA damage which can protect against several other cancer and diseases.

3. Controls Weight: Several sources of carbs like fresh fruits and vegetables can aid in reducing weight if it is followed in a balanced and proportioned diet plan. The appropriate amount and correct choice of carbs intake can help in consuming more fiber which helps in consuming fewer calories only and feeling full for longer periods, thus reducing weight gain.

Proteins

Protein, also known as the building blocks of the body, is another major macronutrient that is made up of the long chains of a compound called amino acids. Protein is crucial for our body as it helps in the repair, growth, development, and maintenance of the tissues in our body. Protein is vital for maintaining the essential functions of our body like improving hormone systems, transport systems, tissue structure, metabolic system, and the enzymes that regulate it, and also to balance the acid/base environment in our body.

The daily intake of protein varies from 0.36 to 1 gram per body weight of an individual but also depends upon how much workout one does. People who indulge in vigorous workouts and exercises can have higher protein safely. One should focus on consuming protein in a proper quantity that can fulfill around 10 to 30% of the calorie intake per day. Our body cannot store protein, so, the body converts the excess protein intake into other forms like fats or energy.

Food Rich in Proteins

Proteins can be easily derived from animals as well as plant-based sources. Animal-based products are the best source of extracting protein through eggs, poultry, seafood, fish, meat, and dairy products. However, processed meat is good in protein content but has saturated fats which makes it an unhealthy choice. Therefore, choosing a protein source must be a wise decision to fulfill the requirement of protein and also extract other benefits. Less known, but several plant sources are also highly rich in protein along with providing other beneficial nutrients like micronutrients and fiber. Some of the rich plant-based sources of protein are whole grains, nuts, seeds, beans, and lentils.

Benefits of Proteins in Diet

1. Reduces Appetite and Controls Weight: Protein is very beneficial for making one feel fuller for longer periods and reduces the craving for hunger or irregular snacking. Protein is known for reducing the level of a hunger hormone called ghrelin and simultaneously works towards boosting the levels of Peptide YY hormone, which can make you feel full for a long time. Therefore, a protein-rich diet can help in controlling weight gain and also reduce some extra kilos, efficiently.

2. Improves Muscle Strength and Increases Mass: Protein is known as the building block of the body as it helps in increasing the mass and strength of the muscle and building tissues. Especially people who perform workouts and vigorous exercises to improve their body mass and build muscle must consume good amounts of protein to achieve the best results.

3. Improves Metabolism and Burns Fats: When we eat any food, our body burns out the calories in the process of digesting food, this is called a thermic effect of food (TEF). Protein has a higher

thermic effect on food when compared with other macronutrients like fats or carbs. Therefore, consuming protein can help in burning out more calories to digest, which is help full for improving the metabolism and can also promote burning fats and reducing weight.

Fats

Fats are another important macronutrient that play a vital role in the body for preserving and storing energy. It is important to consume fats from outside sources as our bodies cannot produce essential fatty acids on their own. One of the key functions of fats is to protect and insulate delicate internal organs. It also assists in the absorption and transportation of several fat-soluble vitamins like A, D E, and K. Fats are categorized into saturated and unsaturated fats based on the impact that they have on our bodies. Saturated fats also called unhealthy fats tend to solidify at room temperature that can get deposited in the blood vessels, causing atherosclerosis, a condition in which arteries get hardened. Consuming saturated fats in excess amounts can increase low-density lipoprotein (LDL), often known as bad cholesterol. High levels of LDL can increase the risk of several types of heart diseases. Unsaturated fats are different from saturated fats in their chemical structure due to which they are in the form of liquid at room temperature. Unsaturated fats are categorized as mono-saturated fats and poly-saturated fats, both of which are good for your health. Therefore, before the consumption of foods rich in fats, you must be aware of the type of fats it contains, to help extract maximum benefits to your health.

Food Rich in Fats

Most healthy types of fats are derived from plant sources also called ploy-saturated and mono-saturated fats. The several important plant sources of unsaturated fats are some kinds of fish like salmon, anchovies, and tuna that contain omega-3 fatty acids, avocados, nuts, olive, and plant-based oil. These fats can be consumed in good amounts so that they do not increase the risk of health issues. However, saturated fats are mostly obtained from the animal sources like meat, lamb, pork, full-fat dairy products, butter, processed meats, and processed and baked food items. So, one must be careful while choosing the source of fats in their diet plan to prevent any harsh consequences on health.

Benefits of Fats in Diet

1. Maintains Cholesterol Levels: Consuming healthy fats in the form of unsaturated or monounsaturated fats can help in maintaining healthy cholesterol levels and improving healthy heart conditions. The most beneficial food items to extract these health benefits can be achieved by consuming fatty fish that are rich in omega-3 fatty acids. Some of these fish are tuna and salmon which can help to attain a healthy heart.

2. Optimizes Brain Function: Unsaturated fats in the form of omega-3 fatty acids are known for their role in improving brain development and boosting the internal mechanism in the brain and reducing the risk of Alzheimer's disease and dementia. Consuming food rich in such fats helps attain good mental health as it can elevate moods and promote a sharp memory.

3. Supports Weight Loss: Unsaturated fats in the form of mono-saturated and ploy-saturated fats help regulate the appetite and also control the release of hunger hormones. Thus, adding a small portion of food products that are rich in healthy fats can

make you feel full for a longer time and reduce the need to eat at shorter intervals or unnecessary snacking. This helps in eating a proportioned diet in a controlled and balanced manner, making it easy to reduce weight and maintain a healthy weight.

Micro Nutrients

Micronutrients are an important group of nutrients that are needed by our body in very small amounts but are extremely important for proper growth, development, and functioning. An imbalance or deficiency of micronutrients can show symptoms of severe health conditions symptoms or even lead to life-threatening situations. One of the main functions of micronutrients is the production of hormones, enzymes, and various other substances that are crucial for the normal growth and nourishment of our body. These nutrients have antioxidant properties and are also responsible for protecting our bodies against several deficiencies and diseases. Our body is incapable of producing these micronutrients on its own, instead, they can be extracted by consuming sources of food that are rich in these vitamins and minerals. Therefore, eating a healthy and diverse diet plan can help in fulfilling the daily requirements of nutrients.

Vitamins

Vitamins are organic substances that are produced either by plants or animals and can be further broken down with the help of air, acid, or heat. Vitamins are classified as water-soluble (like vitamins B and Vitamin C) or fat-soluble (like vitamins A, D E, and K).

Water-Soluble Vitamins

Water-soluble vitamins cannot be stored directly, rather they must be dissolved in water and then absorbed in the body. Consuming higher amounts of water-soluble vitamins could not harm the body as the extra and unused vitamins are lost from the body through urine. Water-soluble vitamins have several important roles in our body which are enlisted in the table below along with their prime food sources:

Water-soluble vitamins	Food Sources	Key Functions
Vitamin B1 (Thiamine)	Fish, whole grains, and meat	Help in converting carbohydrates into energy.
Vitamin B2 (Riboflavin)	Milk, egg, and organ meat	Help in producing energy from proteins by improving cell functioning, aiding in producing red blood cells, and assisting the overall growth of the body.
Vitamin B3 (Niacin)	Beans, salmon, meat, and green leafy vegetables	Help in the metabolism of proteins and fats, converting carbohydrates into glucose, improving nervous system function, and keeping it healthy.
Vitamin B5 (Pantothenic acid)	Avocado, mushrooms, meat, and tuna	Help in synthesizing fatty acids.

Vitamin B6 (Pyridoxine)	Potatoes, milk, carrots, and fish	Help in converting energy by breaking down carbohydrates into glucose and producing red blood cells.
Vitamin B7 (Biotin)	Sweet potatoes, eggs, spinach, and almonds	Help in the metabolism of protein, carbohydrates, and fats.
Vitamin B9 (Folate)	Asparagus, black-eyed peas, spinach, liver, and beef	Aids cell division.
Vitamin B12 (Cobalamin)	Meat, clams, and fish	Help in producing red blood cells and improve the normal functioning of the brain and nervous systems.
Vitamin C (Ascorbic acid)	Brussels Sprouts, Citric fruits, and Bell peppers.	Help in cell protection from free radicals and maintains healthy bones, skin, blood vessels, and cartilage.

Fat-Soluble Vitamins

Fat-soluble vitamins are easily dissolved in the fats, and then they are accumulated in the body. The fat-soluble vitamins are stored in the fatty tissues and liver for further use. Fat-soluble vitamins must not be consumed in excess as it gets highly accumulates in the fats and tissues of the body which can cause hypervitaminosis and toxicity. Several types of fat-soluble vitamins with functions and food sources are listed in the table below:

Fat-Soluble Vitamins	Food Sources	Key Functions
Vitamin A	Carotenoids (spinach, sweet potatoes, and carrots), and retinol (Fish, liver, and dairy)	Improves eyesight, improves immunity, and maintains proper functioning of the liver, heart, and other organs.
Vitamin D	Milk, sunlight, and fish oil	Help in the absorption of calcium and phosphorus which improves none and strengthens them and aids in reducing inflammation.
Vitamin E	Wheat germ, almonds, and sunflower seeds	Work like an antioxidant, which protects the cell from damage and improves the immune system

Vitamin K	Soybeans, pumpkin, and green leafy vegetables	Help in blood clotting and building bones

Minerals

Minerals are the inorganic compounds that are found in the soil, or water, which cannot be further broken down. A mineral present in soil and water is consumed by animals or absorbed by plants. Consuming such plants and animal helps in fulfilling the basic requirements of the important minerals in our body. Each mineral has several important functions for our body that helps in keeping our body healthy. Minerals are categorized as macro minerals and trace minerals:

Macro Minerals

These minerals are needed in larger amounts in our bodies to help them function properly and efficiently. Several important macro minerals and their core functions are listed in the table below:

Macro Minerals	Food Source	Key Functions
Calcium	Broccoli, Green leafy vegetables, and dairy products	Help in keeping bones and teeth healthy, maintain heart rhythm and normal functioning, improve blood clotting, assist in muscle and blood vessel contraction.

Phosphorus	Turkey, salmon, and yogurt	Maintaining an apt level of fluids within the cells, improving muscle contraction, and supporting normal blood pressure.
Magnesium	Black beans, almonds, and cashew	Improves nerve and muscle functioning, regulate blood sugar level and blood pressure, and helps in making bones, protein, and DNA.
Sodium	Canned soups, salt, and processed food items	Conducting nerve impulses that help in the contraction and relaxation of muscles, maintaining an apt balance of minerals and water in the body, and maintaining blood pressure.
Chloride	Celery, seaweed, and salt	Help in maintaining the fluid balance from going in and out of cells, aid in maintaining apt oh level, and stimulating the stomach acids for improving digestion,
Potassium	Acorn squash, lentils, and bananas	Help in regulating the flow of fluids within the cells, maintaining apt blood pressure, and helps in contracting of muscles.

| Sulphur | Mineral water, onions, eggs, garlic, and brussels sprouts | Help in protecting cells from damage, repairing and building DNA, help in producing amino acids, and form the structural component of the exterior layer of human skin. |

Trace Minerals

Trace minerals are required in very fewer amounts by our bodies, but they play a crucial role in keeping our bodies fit and healthy. Trace mineral is the building blocks of various important enzymes in our body which helps in facilitating several biochemical reactions. These minerals have antioxidant properties that improve normal growth and development and also support neurological functions. The important trace mineral along with their key functions and food sources are mentioned in the table below:

Trace Minerals	Food Source	Key Functions
Iron	Spinach, oysters, and white beans	Help boost the functioning of red blood cells that aids in transporting oxygen.
Manganese	Peanuts, pineapples, and pecans	Improve the metabolism of fats, carbs, and protein.

Copper	Cashews, liver, and crabs	Improve the functioning of the brain and nervous system, and supports connective tissue formation.
Zinc	Chickpeas, oysters, and crab	Help in the healing of wounds by improving the immune system and supporting normal growth and development.
Iodine	Yogurt, cod, and seafood	Support regulating thyroids.
Fluoride	Water, fruit juice, and cod	Help in strengthening teeth and bones and preventing decay and weakening.
Selenium	Ham, Brazil nuts, and sardines	Protect against cell damage and infections, supports in making DNA, improving thyroid health, and reproduction.

Chapter 3:

Count Your Calories

To ensure good health: Eat lightly, breathe deeply, live moderately, cultivate cheerfulness and maintain an interest in life. –William Londen, an American Professor

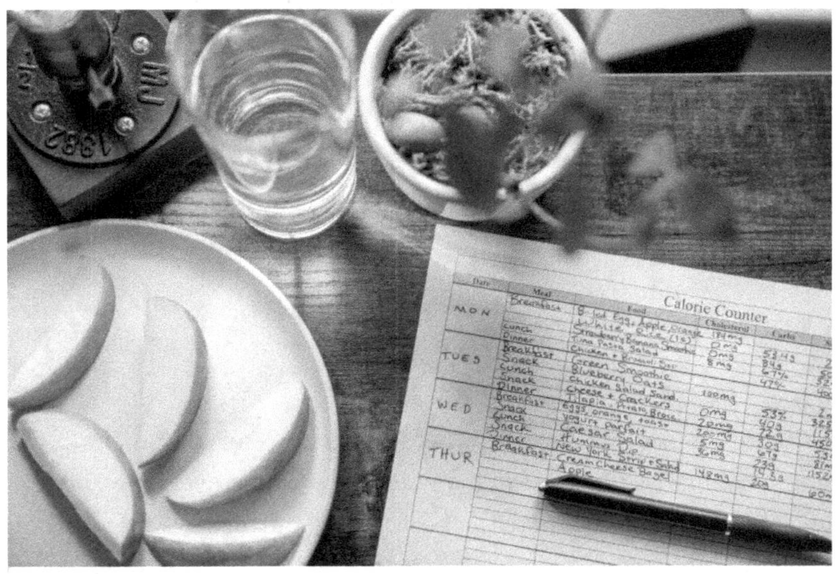

Eating healthy is not just about eating less or following a fixed diet plan, all your life. Instead, it is something more interesting and engrossing, as you gradually learn that each food item that comes before you has a very different story of its composition, which makes it a good or bad choice, in terms of its health parameters. This can be the most challenging part of developing healthy eating habits and prove to be a game-changer in our life, as it can show us the correct way to start working and maintaining our eating patterns. There are various important things that may count while making our diet chart or deciding on which diet plan to follow, like:

- Which is the best food that can help us lower our calorie count?

- How much calorie intake is healthy for us?

- How can we estimate the number of calories in a food item?

- Can checking on our calorie consumption be a helpful step?

- How can we meet our calorie target for the day?

All these mind-boggling questions may create turmoil in your mind and trigger the quest within you, to dive deep into the science of eating healthy and counting your calories, by enjoying your food along with maintaining health and fitness.

What Calories Are?

In scientific terms, a calorie can be defined as a unit that measures the energy content of the food items that we consume every day, which is actually the energy required for performing our daily activities. Thus, consuming the right quantity of calories is vital for our health and survival in this dynamic world, as without sufficient intake of calories the cells in our body would die and this could affect the normal functioning of our heart, lungs, and other important organs, thereby disrupting our overall health. Our body extracts energy from the food we eat in the form of carbohydrates, fats, and proteins. These nutrients are consumed in the form of several sources of foods like carbohydrates can be derived from starches, rice, and sugar.

Calories are important for our body to function and stay active consuming a higher number of calories than what is needed by our body can lead to weight gain and also increases the risk of several diseases. Consuming calories that are optimum for performing every function is the right amount of calories needed by our body to stay healthy and active. Any calorie intake higher or lower than this level would gradually impact our health.

Apart from this, calories are important to understand the potential energy content of each food item that we eat. Calories value is not the same for every food we eat, rather it varies based upon the component of food. The calorie contents of the three most essential food components are:

- One gram of protein has four Kcal

- One gram of carbohydrate has four Kcal

- One gram of fat has nine Kcal

Why Count Your Calories?

Counting calories is a technique that helps in tracking the number of calories that you consume in a day or in a meal that supports maintaining your weight. Counting calories can help you to deal with several health conditions, which can be improved when you change your calorie intake. Health conditions like obesity, chronic heart and cardiovascular diseases, arthritis or joint pains, and several other health conditions need an improvement in your health to lower their impact. In all these cases, counting calories can help in estimating if you are consuming the right type of diet that could improve your health condition. When you track your calorie intake, you can probably make healthy changes in your diet, and limit or exceed the consumption to make yourself more physically fit.

Apart from this counting the calories is a fine way to transform your food consumption patterns towards developing good and healthy eating habits. Counting calories helps in calculating and ensuring that your body is getting the right amount of nutrition. Consuming food without awareness and knowledge about its dietary benefits can lead to malnutrition or even cause overeating, leading to obesity. So, when you count on the calories each time before having meals, you hold yourself accountable for consuming the right food in the right portion that could provide you with several health benefits. The secret behind eating a complete and balanced diet is counting calories.

What is the Ideal Calorie Count?

The first step towards determining the number of calories you should consume in the day needs the recognition of the allowed calorie content per day. The ideal calorie intake varies based on age, gender, health conditions, and physical activities. Having an idea about the above factors makes it easy to choose the right diet that could fulfill the basic calorie requirements for a day. Apart from this, the consumption of calories also depends upon your health conditions, medications (like diabetes medicines or steroids), changing hormones, and your overall health. The recommended guidelines for consuming calories are different for adults, teens, and children, as shown in the table below:

Category	Sub-Category	Calorie/Day
Adults	Men	2.200 to 3,200 calories per day
	Women	1,600 to 2,400 calories per day
Teenagers	Boys	1,600 to 2,200 calories per day
	Girls	2,000 to 2,600 calories per day

It is easy to lose weight if you simply rely upon the ideal calorie intake recommended values. While consuming a diet that is not rich in nutrition could make the journey of losing weight quite challenging. Eating a less nutritious diet also increases the chances of overeating and feeling hungry frequently. Furthermore, eating an empty-calorie diet could do no benefit as it lacks the helpful nutrition that may support an active and healthy lifestyle. So, to reach the goal of achieving good health it is important to eat a nutritious diet that could make you feel energetic, strong, and satiated. Therefore, having an idea about the calorie content of various food items can help improve your meal plans and achieve good health. So, let's have a look at the calories present in various common food items, which can help you to consume a balanced diet.

How to Count Your Calorie Intake?

Counting calories is a valuable technique that helps to reach the milestones of weight loss, weight gain or just maintaining a healthy weight. For evaluating the number of calories you intake, it is important to first calculate the daily requirement of calories by your body to maintain the current weight. This can be calculated through simple mathematics, multiply your current weight (in pounds only) by 15 to get a rough estimate of the number of calories your body is consuming for maintaining this weight. Now, based on the weight and calorie intake, you can decide how many calories to cut down to reduce the extra weight. On average for reducing 1 to 2 pounds every week, one must cut down 500 to 1000 calories per day. This must be followed by a vigorous 30-minute workout or simply by exercising at home. However, one must be careful while reducing the amount of calorie intake, as it can impact one's health since the body is not habitual to the change in the quantities of various important nutrients. Experts have revealed that the minimum calorie intake for women must not fall below 1200 calories per day, while for men the minimum level is approximately 1500 calories per day.

Another important step in counting calories is choosing your meal plans that can help meet your daily target of calories. One easy approach to counting the calories is to check the number of calories present in the food and then design your menu plan. The calories present in the most common food items are enlisted below, which can help you to wisely decide upon your meals for the day and stay healthy:

Food Items	Serving Size	Calories
Breads		
Regular Bread	One Slice	60-80
French Bread	One Slice	60-80
Whole-Wheat Bagel	One Piece	360
Plain Bagel	One Piece	320
Pita Bread	One Piece	150
English Muffins	One Piece	135
Cereals		
Cornflakes	One Cup	100
All Bran	Half Cup	79
Rolled Oats	One Cup	145
Rice Krispies	One Cup	98
Fruits		

Apple	One Piece	95
Banana	One Piece	110
Mango	One Cup (sliced)	122
Grapes	One Cup	104
Strawberries	One Cup (sliced)	53
Watermelon	One Cup (diced)	46
Papaya	One Cup	71
Blueberries	One Cup	84
Peaches	One Piece	63
Kiwi	One Piece	50
Avocado	One Slice	24
Cherries	One Piece	4.4
Vegetables		

Carrot	One Piece (medium)	25
Potato	One Skin	22
Tomato	One Cup	32
Beetroot	One Piece	50
Broccoli	One Cup	31
Dairy Products		
Milk	One Cup	146
Yogurt	One Cup	149
Cream	One Cup	809
Cottage Cheese	One Cup	300
Cream Cheese	One Cup	812
Cheddar Cheese	One Cup	532
Mozzarella Cheese	One Cup	335
Butter	One Pat	36

Butter Milk	One Cup	151
Beverages		
Tea	One Cup	120
Green Tea	One Cup	2.4
Black Tea	One Cup	2.4
Coffee with Milk	One Cup	82
Black Coffee	One Cup	2.4
Aeriated Drinks	One Can	156
Beer	One Can	155
Poultry		
Chicken	100 gm	143
Boiled Egg	One Piece	72
Fried Egg	One Piece	90
Poached Egg	One Piece	72

	Meat	
Red Meat	100 gm	282
White Meat	100 gm	188
	Seafood	
Fried Fish	One Filet	199
Baked Fish	One Filet	111
Steamed Fish	One Filet	157
	Junk Food	
Pizza	One Piece	406
Burger	One Piece	254
Fries	Medium	378
Patties	One Patty	94
Noodles	One Cup	219
Hot Dog Sandwich	One Piece	123

Sweets		
Pastries	One Piece	307
Ice creams	One Cup	279
Frozen Yogurt	One Cup	222
Brownies	100 gm	434
Custard	One Cup	247
Donuts	**One Piece**	260
Cinnamon Rolls	**One roll**	115

If calculating calories every day is a tiring task for you, then another different approach is to restrict the number of calories you consume. This can be easily done by cutting down the intake of food having higher calories, instead of choosing meals with fewer calories. Cutting down the calories alone could not bring the change, rather you must focus on an appropriate eating schedule that helps in eating a complete but portioned meal at certain times of the day, helping you to achieve your goals efficiently. While the entire process of counting calories is quite simple, doing some common blunders could interrupt the path to success. Following a few interesting and simple calorie counting tips given below could probably help one in avoiding common mistakes and improve the results:

1. Use new and advanced technical tools like advanced applications for instant calorie calculation. Simply relying on memory

increases the chances of errors, as it is difficult to remember the exact and accurate intake of the calories. Thus, a calorie-tracking application could solve this issue.

2. You must be careful in measuring the portion of each meal accurately. Don't do the guesswork to determine the size or quantity of the meal. Instead, it is recommended to use standard measuring cups or kitchen digital scales to help in measuring the exact portion of food that you consume. This could help in evaluating the correct amount of calorie intake.

3. Another important point is to stay within your budget. It is not mandatory to spend a lot on buying a tool or a gadget for counting your calories. You can easily find several options for counting calories be it online, with any gadget, or simply the traditional ways of writing on paper. If you are working on a computer the whole day, then using an online application could be a better option. Otherwise, chose a small notepad or small notebook to jot down the calories.

4. One thing that most of us forget is to note down the number of other nutrients that we consume and also the physical activities that we do in a complete day. Apart from calculating calories, counting on the macros and physical workouts also helps in getting precise results that would ease the process of reaching your goal.

Advanced Calorie Counting Apps

In a dynamically mechanized world, where doing every other task is made easy with the help of advanced technology, similarly, several new applications have evolved that have made counting calories just a click away. The calorie counter apps are a great and helpful tool that helps in analyzing and estimating the daily calorie intake without any hassle. These calorie counting applications are not only helpful for reducing weight but also promote giving up the bad habits of unhealthy snacking and eating at irregular intervals of time, which helps in boosting overall health. Apart from indicating the maximum intake of calories per day, a calorie counter app also helps in realizing if the food intake is too less. Eating very less food can cause a slowdown in the resting metabolic rate, which prevents excessive weight loss and initiates weight regain. Further, a calorie counter is the best way to improve consistency, as self-tracking the calories inculcate a sense of accountability which is the fundamental factor to gaining success in the endeavor of weight loss.

Out of the availability of wide options for choosing a calorie counter, there are a few important points that could help in selecting the best one. Some of these points of consideration are user ratings, transparency about subscriptions, bills and personal information, features, price, and user reviews. Popular calorie counter apps are Cronometer, My Fitness Pal, Noom, Lifesum, My Net Diary, Fat Secret, and Lose It! The special features of a few commonly preferred apps are discussed below:

1. My Fitness Pal: It is an easy, popular, and high-rated calorie counter application that has its basic version available for free, while the advanced versions cost $19.99 per month or $79.99 for 1 year. Apart from calculating the daily calorie intake, it also has an exercise log and a food diary which has more than 11 million food enlisted. The home page is well designed that shows the amount of calorie intake for a day along with the physical exercises performed, helping in calculating the calories consumed and burnt for a day.

2. Lose It!: This calorie counter is known for its personalized recommendation of calorie intake based on weight, age, height, and goals. The basic version of this app is available for free use,

while the premium version is available for only $39.99 per year. This app has a feature to save the common recipes for later entry and also scans the barcode of packaged food items for easy calculation of calories. This app presents weight loss in the form of a graph and also has the option of active live chat for instant help and advice.

3. Fat Secret: This app is free for all users and has various features like a food diary, exercise log, nutrition database, weight chart, bar code scanner, and journal. The best thing about this app is that it shows a summary of the monthly consumption of calories which is good for tracking the progress. Along with the basic features, this app has a community chat where users can share new recipes, success stories, and helpful tips. Apart from this, a feature called "Challenges" helps in creating or participating in a closed group to share and discuss dietary problems and their solutions.

Benefits to Count Your Calories

One question that keeps hovering in our mind, every time we think about losing weight is to count the calorie intake. The concept of developing a healthy lifestyle is often preoccupied with the notions of cutting down on calorie intake and practically giving up everything that we love to eat. However, counting calories is not all about only shedding some extra kilos, rather it is an effortful step to stay healthy. Being calorie deficient is not a good sign of leading healthy life. So, let's explore the magical power of counting calories in maintaining a healthy body:

1. Improves your Food Choices: Beginning the journey of counting calories for everything that you eat can help in improving your knowledge and awareness about the food items that are healthy

and unhealthy for your body. It is a common habit among most of us to eat just anything and everything, without even being thoughtful about its nutritional value and calorie count. However, once you start to check out on the calories, the eagerness and enthusiasm to opt for healthier food choices would become a priority. This could help in being accountable to yourself and keeping track to progress better.

2. Focuses on Eating Smaller Portions: Controlling calorie intake is not about restricting several food items, rather it is more about being conscious of eating the right amount of healthy food at the proper time. It's not an easy task to give up your favorite food. Calorie counting does not restrict any type of food, rather it is the best and most feasible way to cut down and focus on consuming a more portioned diet, which is full of nutrition and health benefits. Paying attention to the calories present in each food item helps in visualizing the benefits of a healthy portioned diet, which also gives you a chance to eat your favorite meals but in a controlled manner.

3. Aids in a Healthy Weight Loss Process: The entire process of losing some extra kilos is about consuming a diet that has fewer calories, which is followed by a regular exercise routine to burn the extra calories. In this endeavor, counting on the calories act like a morale booster that motivates and eases the weight loss struggle. Counting the calories can help you to analyze and estimate the calories you have eaten in a day and predict your weight loss progress.

4. Creates Motivation by Visualizing Your Meal: Achieving success in any sphere of life is hidden in our subconscious mind. Similarly, is the case when you decide to work towards improving your health and try to shed some weight. Counting calories helps in visualizing your progress, as when you see it, you can work

better towards your goal. It empowers you by inculcating the enthusiasm and eagerness to continue on the journey of weight loss and make yourself healthier.

Chapter 4:

Best Diet Plans to Stay Healthy

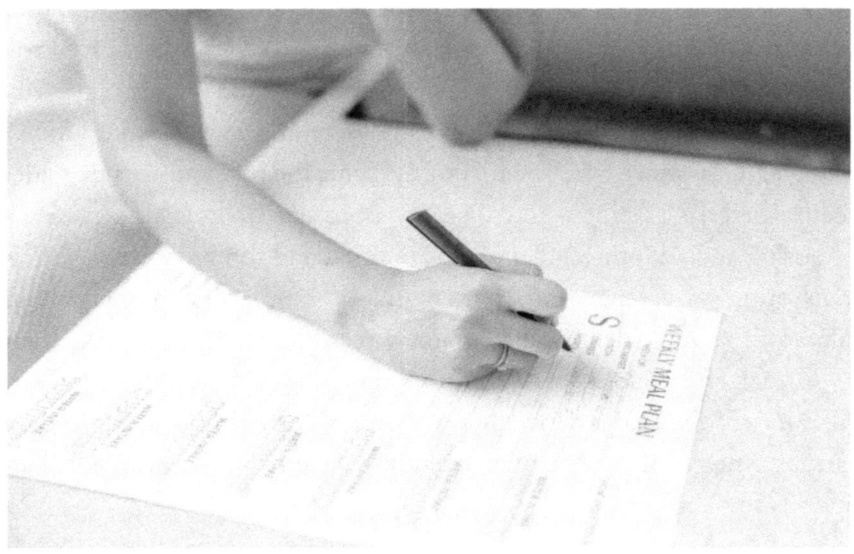

Relating to the famous quote mentioned above by Denis Waitley, an American motivational speaker who has emphasized the importance of health and has correlated it with time. However, we are all well aware that lost time is never found and despite being aware of all the worldly facts, we still tend to commit the biggest mistakes of our life when we knowingly or unknowingly overlook the importance of our health and eating a good and balanced diet. Often preoccupied to maintain a good balance between our professional and personal fronts, one tends to ignore their health. One of the most common and negative habits found among us is that until we lose our health, we never understand its importance. By the time, we realize the significance of achieving a healthy lifestyle it is often too late as the adopted bad habits of eating, sleeping, and lower physical activities instill their strong place in our life. In other words, these unhealthy dietary and eating habits bind in their magical spell, enslaving us, which makes it a challenging task to overcome those habits. In fact, in some cases, we only get to understand and value our health once we are unwell and begin to see the symptoms of several kinds of chronic health diseases, diabetes or obesity, etc.

Good health is one of the biggest achievements in one's life and putting in useful efforts to develop supportive eating habits can play a vital role in avoiding harsh consequences. Amongst the several major inputs, one of the best investments would be to analyze and evaluate the kind of eating habits that we follow. Most of the time, the root cause of degraded health, diverse illnesses, and diseases is related to our diet patterns. Choosing and adopting a diet plan is the first and foremost step towards transforming ourselves into better and healthier versions. There are numerous kinds of diets available that we can choose from, each of them is distinct and unique from one another, based upon the type and quantity of food that is allowed to eat. So, let's dive deep and explore the various types of diet plans that would provide us with a wide idea and options to choose from.

Low-Carb Diet

A low-carb diet is famous for reducing weight naturally without the need to skip meals or avoid any kind of food that is known for its nutritional value. As the name suggests, a low-carb diet plan emphasizes consuming a healthy and nutritious diet plan but cutting down the intake of a significant amount of carbohydrates. The most common types of food items that have higher carbohydrates like starchy vegetables, fruits, and grains are limited to a certain extent. A low-carb diet is categorized into many other types which are differentiated based on the number of carbs that are allowed per day. Some of the famous low-carb diets are:

Types	Specifications
Ketogenic or Keto Diet	The allowed percentage of carbs per day is less than 10% which ranges from 20 to 50 grams per day.
Atkins Diet	At the initial stage, the allowed percentage of carbs is less than 10% (20- to 40 grams per day), while in later stages the allowed percentage of carbs is less than 20% approximating less than 100 grams per day.
South Beach Diet	Allows the consumption of lean meat and heart-healthy fatty foods. In the initial stages the intake of fruits is limited, while in the 2nd and 3rd phases of this diet plan, these restricted food items can be added back.
Paleo Diet	A naturally low-carb diet restricts the intake of diverse carbs sources like legumes, grains, and dairy products. While the complete focus is on consuming fresh meats, vegetables, and fruits.
Dukan Diet	A restrictive eating plan that emphasizes a higher intake of protein and a lower intake of fats.

A simple low-carb diet plan stresses the consumption of protein-rich food and non-starchy vegetables that can help in achieving the daily nutrient requirement. Most food items that are strictly restricted are pasta, bread, starchy vegetables, grains, and legumes. While adopting this plan, one can consume lean meats, low-carb fruits, non-starchy vegetables, nuts, seeds, full dairy products, oils, fats, and fish. Following this diet plan does not completely limit the intake of restricted food items. However, munching on your favorite fruit, snacks, or sweetened beverages only on an occasional basis is allowed. The flexibility allowance in a low-carb diet makes it quite easy and feasible for one to follow and stick to it, working towards their goal of achieving good health.

Ketogenic Diet

When you are bothered about losing weight too quickly or struggling to shed some extra fats from your body, you can definitely think of the ketogenic diet plan, without any doubt. A simple ketogenic diet works majorly by restricting the intake of carbohydrates from our diet and replacing it with food items rich in fats and proteins, in order to initiate the process of ketosis. The term ketosis may sound new to many of us, but it explains the science behind the working of a ketogenic diet. What actually happens is, when we stop eating carbohydrate rich-food, our body consumes all the stored carbohydrates slowly and in a span of 3-4 days, all these stored carbohydrates get over. This drives our body to start utilizing the stored fats and proteins in it, in order to generate energy, to do work. This natural process of switching the body's fuel from carbohydrates to fats or proteins is scientifically termed ketosis. Thus, the main idea behind adopting a ketogenic diet is to reduce some extra kilos in very less time to achieve better health, without disrupting our meal cycles.

Moreover, during the course of this diet, our body produces ketones, which are released as a result of the breakdown of fats which act as energy providers for the body in a keto diet plan. In a ketogenic diet, the minimum recommended quantity of carbohydrate intake is less than 50 grams per day, or in some cases even less than 20 grams. A ketogenic diet is called a low-carb diet also, with many similarities with the Atkins diet, and can be practiced in different forms like a standard ketogenic diet and high protein ketogenic diet which are generally followed by most people. Other variations of the ketogenic diet include the cyclical ketogenic diet and targeted ketogenic diet which is mostly preferred by athletes, weight lifters, and bodybuilders for more noticeable and long-term results.

Here, we have a sorted list of all the food items that can be consumed by you without giving a second thought, during the journey through your ketogenic diet:

1. Animal protein—seafood, fish, meat, poultry, and egg.

2. Dairy products—all types of cheese, plain Greek yogurt, milk cream, cottage cheese, etc.

3. Unsweetened plant-based milk—soy milk, coconut milk, etc.

4. Vegetables—all types of green leafy vegetables, peppers, high-fat vegetables like avocado, summer squash like zucchini and yellow squash, and any non-starchy vegetable.

5. Plant-based food—nuts, seeds, berries, dark chocolate, and cocoa powder.

6. Fats and oils—olive oil, ghee, butter, avocado oil, and coconut oil.

7. Beverages—unsweetened tea and coffee.

Apart from these, there is also a long list of food items that must be strictly avoided when you are following a ketogenic diet, for achieving quick and effective results. For instance, sweet potatoes, potatoes, beetroot, corn, onion, grains, legumes, fruits, sweetened beverages, sugar drinks, candy, and various sauces that contain sugar. On the whole, anything that is rich in sugar is to be avoided, so that we can set a regular and healthy eating habit with a keto diet plan.

Simple Diet Plans

Moreover, here we have a very helpful and delicious two-day meal chart so that you can easily enjoy the perks of a ketogenic diet by including it in your daily routine:

	Day-1	Day-2
Breakfast	• Mushroom omelet	• Almond milk smoothies with favorite greens, protein powder, and almond butter
Morning snacks	• Sunflower seeds	• Plain Greek yogurt
Lunch	• Grilled beef kebabs with sautéed vegetables	• Grilled salmon with green salad
Evening Snacks	• Celery sticks with almond butter	• Kale chips
Dinner	• Zucchini noodles with added meatballs and cream sauce topping	• Roasted chicken with sautéed green vegetables

Health Benefits

Adopting a ketogenic diet may initially seem to be a challenge for many of you but believe me when you will ponder over the positive changes it will bring about in your life you will indeed get motivated to get going with this awesome diet plan. A ketogenic diet basically focuses on reducing the consumption of food items that are rich in carbohydrates thereby increasing the intake of fats which are helpful in utilizing the ketones in our body, in order to provide energy for the proper functioning of the body. On the brighter side, this process aids in burning the excess fats stored in our body and thus promotes efficient weight loss. One of the biggest advantages of a ketogenic diet is that the food products that are consumed can help us in feeling full for a longer period which automatically reduces hunger and unnecessary craving and munching on food items that have higher calories in them. However, a ketogenic diet plan demands strict adherence to eating habits, making it quite challenging to stick to it for a longer time.

A ketogenic eating plan is an effective strategy for all those who suffer from type-1 and type-2 diabetes, as it strictly restricts the consumption of food items rich in sugar or any type of sweetened beverages that eventually help to manage and control the blood sugar level in our body with ease. However, following this eating plan for longer could lead to hypoglycemia or low blood sugar level. Hence, it is recommended that anyone with severe health conditions should consult their healthcare provider and get a clear picture of the pros and cons of a ketogenic diet plan, before switching to it for the long term.

Atkins Diet

Atkins diet is also one of the best eating plans that can help in natural weight loss, without even the need to count up on the calories. Following an Atkins diet plan emphasizes the intake of food that are low in carbs but higher in protein or fat intake. A diet plan that is rich in protein consumption can help in reducing the appetite, as you may feel full for longer periods of time. This helps in reducing the urge to hunger and other unnecessary snacking. This diet plan is a four-phase phenomenon that happens one after another.

Induction Phase (Phase-1)—The initial phase stresses consuming less than 20 grams of carbs for at least 2 weeks regularly. In these 14 days, one must eat foods rich in protein and fats, and low carbs green vegetables only, which may help to trigger weight loss.

Balancing Phase (Phase-2)—Gradually after phase-1, start adding more nuts, small amounts of fruits, and other low-carb vegetables to your diet.

Fine-Tuning Phase (Phase-3)—This phase begins when you have almost reached near to your goal weight. At this point in time, begin adding some more carbs to your diet plan until the weight loss slows down.

Maintenance Phase (Phase-4)—This is the most important phase, as you can begin eating all types of healthy carbs which your body can easily retain without regaining back some extra weight.

These phases form an important part of the Atkins diet as it helps in creating balance in the body, ensuring to provide all the necessary nutrient to the body which is essential for healthy growth and lifestyle. However, one can stick to any single phase for longer periods of time, depending upon the need of the body. Several food items that can be consumed during this diet plan are low-carb vegetables, meats, eggs, full-fat dairy products, healthy fats, nuts, seeds, seafood, and fish. Furthermore, the several food items that must be avoided during this diet are high-carb vegetables, grains, sugar, starches, and legumes. However, one can start consuming legumes, high-carb vegetables, and starches once the induction phase is over. Apart from this, beverages like coffee, green tea, and water can be consumed during this diet plan in all phases, without any concern for weight gain.

Sample Meal Plans

	Day-1	Day-2
Breakfast	• Omelet and low-carb vegetables fried in coconut oil	• Bacon and egg
Morning Snacks	• A handful of walnuts	• One or Two slices of cheese
Lunch	• Tuna salad with olive oil	• Grilled chicken with green vegetables and salsa
Evening Snacks	• One cup Greek yogurt with nuts	• One or two hard-boiled eggs
Dinner	• Cheeseburger with green leafy vegetables, butter, and without any bun	• Fried salmon and low-carb vegetables in butter

Health Benefits

As the Atkins diet plan is specially designed to reduce the excess weight from the body, it serves the benefits like reduced risk of heart disease, cardiovascular diseases, and diabetes. Also, a diet plan that helps in reducing weight is naturally beneficial to improve blood pressure and lowers cholesterols levels, while in some cases it may only work temporarily. However, curbing the normal diet plan into the early phase can lead to show some symptoms of headaches, dizziness, constipation, fatigue, and weakness, but these symptoms may subside as the body prolongs adopting this eating plan. Also, anyone who is taking oral diabetes or insulin medications, or suffering from severe kidney disorder must consult a health care professional before switching to this diet plan to avoid serious side effects.

South Beach Diet

A south beach diet is a type of low-carb diet that promotes the intake of unsaturated fats, lean meat, and low-glycemic index carb. The main purpose of this diet is to reduce the consumption of saturated fats which can impact heart health if consumed for longer periods. Apart from this, the south beach diet also stresses including high-fiber fruits and vegetables, which may be having high carbs as well. This eating plan is comprised of healthy fats, complex carbs, and lean protein, which aids in fulfilling the daily requirement of fiber and nutrients in our body that makes it a fit for lifetime consumption and maintaining good health. Food items rich in good crabs include all varieties of fruits, vegetables, legumes, beans, and vegetables. While the intake of bad carbs s completely restricted like refined sugar, refined white flour, and baked food products are.

This diet plan is a three-phase diet plan, the first and second phases emphasize weight loss, while the last phase helps maintain weight. Unlike a strict low-carb diet in which the allowed carbs per day are very low like 20 to 40 grams only, a south beach diet plan allows an intake of 140 grams of carbs in its third phase. Apart from this, this eating plan also emphasizes doing regular exercises that can help in v-boosting the metabolism and avoiding the condition of weight loss plateau. So, let's explore the three phases of the south beach diet plan:

Phase-1—In this initial phase, you must cut down on the consumption of any types of saturated fats, sugar, and all sources of carbohydrates like pasta, grains, fruit, or rice. This phase must be followed strictly for at least 2 weeks regularly which stresses consuming only lean protein like soy products, seafood, lean beef, and skinless poultry. Apart from this, during this phase, you can also consume low-fat dairy products, high-fiber vegetables, seeds, nuts, and avocados.

Phase-2—This is a longer phase as compared to phase-1 and can be continued till you successfully reach your goal weight. During this phase, one can begin gradually to consume several food products that were restricted during phase-1 like brown rice fresh fruits and vegetables, whole grains, and whole wheat pasta.

Phase-3—Also known as the maintenance phase, it is the most important one, as you have to control your new reduced weight, while you are allowed to eat all food items that are allowed in the above phases, but only in moderation.

Sample Meal Plans

	Day-1	Day-2
Breakfast	• Omelet with low-carb vegetables and smoked salmon along with tea	• Baked eggs with green leafy vegetables and chicken slice with coffee
Morning Snacks	• Roasted chickpeas	• Chilled espresso custard
Lunch	• Tuna salad along with coffee	• Grilled Tuna or chicken with grilled vegetable
Evening Snacks	• Celery sticks with peanut butter	• Cottage cheese with sliced bell pepper
Dinner	• Grilled chicken with grilled vegetables and salad	• Vegetables salad with shrimps

Health Benefits

Like any other low-carb diet, this diet plan is also the best for natural weight loss. A higher intake of protein-rich food helps in subsiding hunger which makes it easy for one to stick to an eating plan for longer durations, easing weight loss. Apart from this, consuming food items with low saturated fats reduces the risk of increased cholesterol levels which helps in improving heart health.

Paleo Diet

The Paleo diet is an amazing diet plan that is derived from the food intake habits of ancient people belonging to the Paleo thoric era that existed about 2.5 million to 10,000 years ago. These people in the past used to go hunting to find their food, full of nutrition like fresh vegetables, fruits, fish, lean, meat, eggs, and nuts. Sometimes, this diet plan is also referred to as the Stone Age diet, plethoric diet, Hunter diet, or Caveman diet. Nowadays, the diet followed by most people is full of processed foods, extra sugar, and grains which are produced through farming and are regarded as the new eating habits. While our body is not able to adopt these new and other eating habits that become the root cause of several illnesses and diseases. This mismatch of the new eating habits and the basic body requirements increases the risk of several heart diseases like strokes and cancers, obesity, and increased risk of diabetes. Therefore, the Paleo diet plan guides a person to eat food that is suitable for their body and avoid most food items like processed foods, fatty dairy products, and various kinds of grains.

Several food items that form the main part of a Paleo diet include fresh fruits, vegetables, lean meats, several kinds of seafood, and fish especially the ones rich in omega-3 acid. This diet plan also allows you to consume eggs, nuts seeds, and oils derived from fruits and nuts like olive oil and walnut oil. While, a Paleo diet plans strictly restricts the intake of a list of food items, for instance:

- All processed food items like fries, muffins, and cookies

- All types of grains like wheat, barley, and rye,

- Several types of legumes like beans, lentils, and peanuts.

- All the starchy vegetables like sweet potato, corn, peas, and potato

- Dairy products like milk and cheese

- Added sugar and excess salt

So, a Paleo diet is a proven healthy choice as it helps in consuming the important nutrients, minerals, and vitamins that are essential for healthy growth and nourishment of the body.

Sample Diet Plans

	Day-1	Day-2
Breakfast	• Omelet with green vegetables and mushrooms	• Two Scrambled eggs with Spinach and tomatoes
Morning Snacks	• Ten almonds	• One orange
Lunch	• Roasted chicken with fresh green salad in olive oil dressing	• Salmon fried in butter with green vegetables and tomatoes
Evening Snacks	• One sliced apple with sprinkled cinnamon	• Diced bananas topped with blueberries and nuts

<table>
<tr><td>Dinner</td><td>• Tuna salad in olive oil dressing</td><td>• Beef stir-fried in butter or olive oil with green vegetables</td></tr>
</table>

Health Benefits

A Paleo diet is based upon consuming fresh fruits and vegetables which helps in acquiring the key nutrients required for healthy growth of the body and reducing the risk of several health disorders and illnesses. The restricted intake of refined sugar, fatty dairy products, and processed food items aid in natural weight loss and maintaining a healthy weight, diminishing the chances of obesity. This diet plan reduces the intake of salt which is also helpful to maintain blood pressure and manage cholesterol levels and triglycerides which reduces the chances of increased heart diseases and reduces the risk of heart attacks and cancers.

A Paleo diet is a good choice for maintaining a healthy lifestyle if the allowed food items are consumed in a balanced manner which helps in fulfilling the complete daily requirements of nutrients for the body. However, the restricted intake of several types of grains and legumes can raise doubts about their nutritional value. Grains and legumes are considered rich sources of protein, fiber, and other nutrients. Therefore, to ensure the daily nutritional requirements, one must strictly follow this diet plan in a balanced way and achieve a healthier lifestyle.

Dukan Diet

A Dukan diet is a highly restrictive and strict diet plan that encourages the intake of a high-protein and low-carb diet. In the early phases of this diet, the daily intake of carbs is limited to 20 to 40 grams only which makes it very challenging for one to follow regularly. This diet plan includes the consumption of oat bran as one of the daily nutritional supplements. This diet has 4 phases out of which the first phase has low flexibility of allowed foods, but this diet truly proves to show great results. At the beginning of the diet plan, you calculate your goal weight which is called 'true weight'. To reach this true weight, any of the four phases must not be avoided which will yield quick and effective results.

Attack Phase (Phase-1)—This phase begins with calculating the truer weight and consuming only protein food items and 1.5 tablespoons of oat bran every day as a supplement. This phase lasts for about 1 week only.

Cruise Phase (Phase-2)—This phase can be followed for 1 month or 12 months depending upon the requirement of your body to see visible weight loss results. This diet allows the intake of alternate lean protein for one day, followed by a non-starchy vegetable and lean protein the next day. While it is necessary to consume 2 tablespoons of oat bran every day.

Consolidation Phase (Phase-3)—This is the most special phase, as it is followed for five days when each time 1 pound of weight is lost during the above two phases. This phase allows eating lots of vegetables, protein, some types of fats, and carbs, along with 2.5 tablespoons of oat brans every day.

Stabilization Phase (Phase-4)—This phase is indefinite and can last for as much as you want but only if the true weight is achieved. This phase allows relaxation of the strict food limits followed in the above three phases while consuming three tablespoons of oat bran every day.

Sample Meal Plans

	Day-1	Day-2
Breakfast	• Scrambled eggs with low-fat cheese	• Turkey slices with low-fat cream cheese
Morning Snacks	• Oat bran muffins with tea	• Low-fat yogurt
Lunch	• Grilled Beef with low-fat yogurt	• Chicken curry
Evening Snacks	• Celery sticks with peanut butter	• Oat bran pancakes with coffee
Dinner	• Steamed salmon with herbs	• Baked chicken meatballs

Health Benefits

A Dukan diet is best for anyone who is suffering from a kind of health disorder, as it is a highly restrictive diet. The best advantage of following a Dukan diet is the promising weight loss if followed regularly and consistently. This diet also cuts down any type of saturated food and refined sugar that can help in reducing the risk of heart and cardiovascular diseases. However, if you are facing any serious health issues like diabetes or blood pressure, then it is recommended to consult a healthcare professional before adopting this diet plan.

Intermittent Diet

More than 60 years ago, maintaining weight was an easy task as the people at that time mostly followed an active lifestyle and healthy eating habits. There were no facilities for computers, TV shows were limited to a maximum of 11 p.m. and people followed a disciplined habit of going early to bed. The most common recreational activities were playing outdoors, going out to meet friends, and engaging in several indoor and outdoor physical activities. However, with the emergence of new technology, the habit of mortals has changed drastically. Nowadays, we usually spend most of our time sitting at our home idol, watching our favorite TV shows for longer duration followed by unhealthy snacking. Moreover, with the emergence of technology, access to entertainment activities through TV and the internet is available 24x7 which has disturbed sleeping patterns. This unhealthy living style has emerged as the root cause of several chronic heart diseases like strokes and heart attacks, increased risk of type 2 diabetes, obesity, and other illness.

Diet is one of the first and foremost steps that can help us to correct our bad habits and transform our lifestyles into better ones. An intermittent diet is one such diet plan that can easily support maintaining a healthy weight and even supports weight loss. This diet plan means that you do not eat or keep a fast for a certain period each day or every alternate day or every week. There are several ways to follow an intermittent diet plan:

- Keeping a fast on alternate days. This type of intermittent fasting requires one to eat a complete meal on one day, then switch to complete fasting or consume a meal with less than 500 grams of calorie intake on the next day.

- Keeping a 5:2 fasting requires eating a full complete meal 5 days a week and fasting for the next 2 days a week.

- Everyday time-restricted fasting focuses on eating all types of food for a fixed 8 hours span in the day. For instance, you can skip your breakfast and have your lunch and dinner included in the span of 8 hours every day at the same time.

Intermittent fasting restricts food intake for several hours or days, which helps in exhausting the limit of glucose in our body to produce energy. Rather the body begins to burn out the stored fats for providing energy, leading to metabolic switching. Adapting to this diet plan, strictly limits the intake of food items that are rich in calories like processed foods, refined sugar, and other sweetened beverages. However, during the time of fasting, you can consume several drinks throughout the day that can help to keep yourself hydrated and fresh like water and black coffee which have zero calories. Other food items that can be consumed during this type of eating plan include green leafy vegetables, lean protein, whole grains, and healthy fats.

Sample Diet Plans

	Day-1	Day-2	Day-3
Breakfast	• Multigrain bread sandwich with one egg and green vegetables	• Black Coffee	• Pancakes
Morning Snacks	• One orange	• Water	• One apple
Lunch	• Hummus with falafel rolls	• Tea	• Brown rice with chicken or beef
Afternoon Snacks	• Greek Yogurt with chia seeds or nuts	• Water	• Green smoothie
Dinner	• Grilled chicken with a green salad	• Herbal Tea	• Tuna salad

Health Benefits

An intermittent diet can have a positive impact on your health if it is followed regularly and properly daily. One of the most important benefits f this diet plan is that it supports maintaining good health. Losing extra calories and ability to maintain an active lifestyle can assist in reducing the risk of obesity, diabetes, several cancers, and sleep apnea. This diet plan is also helpful in reducing the diseases that show the symptoms of inflammation, for instance, strokes, asthma, multiple sclerosis, Alzheimer's disease arthritis, etc.

However, switching to an intermittent diet plan may have side effects on your health in the initial phases like nausea, fatigue, insomnia, hunger, and headaches. With consistent practice and following this diet plan regularly, the body gradually adapts to this eating plan, gradually reducing these negative symptoms over a month. This eating plan is recommended for a healthy being, but anyone going through health conditions like pregnancy, gastroesophageal reflux, diabetes, or kidney stones must consult their healthcare physician before switching to this eating plan.

Mediterranean Diet

A Mediterranean diet is acclaimed as one of the world's best eating plans due to its phenomenal impact on the body improves physical health, boosts cognitive and mental health aids in increasing lifespans, and reduces the risk of several diseases. Often regarded as the 'Gold Standard' a Mediterranean diet is valued for providing complete nutrition and sustainable health benefits.

This diet plan is inspired by the common way of eating habits in Mediterranean countries like Spain, Greece, Italy, and Turkey, which is based on higher consumption of fresh fruits, vegetables, legumes, whole grains, and lean meats. This eating habit emphasizes the importance of intake of nuts, seeds, and oils like olive oil in good quantity, and is mostly included as a part of every meal. However, the intake of red meat is completely restricted, while it allows the consumption of dairy products, eggs, and poultry on rare occasions and in moderate amounts only. Due to the negative impact on health, the intake of refined sugar, refined grains, highly processed foods, and processed meats is not allowed. In simple words, a Mediterranean diet is more about consuming quality food products rather than focusing on any single type of food, which aims at providing a quality lifestyle.

Sample Diet Plans

	Day-1	Day-2
Breakfast	• Poached egg with baked sweet potato	• Chia pudding topped with walnuts and blueberries
Morning Snacks	• One orange	• Three plums
Lunch	• Falafel rolls in pita bread, hummus topped with olive oil and green salad	• Grilled chicken with fresh green salad in an olive oil dressing
Evening Snacks	• One carrot, half beetroot with two tbsp. hummus	• One cup of raspberries with half a cup of Greek yogurt
Dinner	• One and a half cups of chicken with vegetable soup	• Fish baked with garlic and basil leaves with quinoa salad

Health Benefits

A Mediterranean diet plan is not a calorie-restricted eating plan, rather it is known for consuming fresh fruits, vegetables, legumes, nuts, and grains with a liberal intake of olive oil and a moderate amount of dairy products and red meat. The followers of the Mediterranean diet plan automatically reduce the intake of saturated fats, processed food, refined sugar, and salt which reduces the risk of several types of heart diseases and helps fight obesity and diabetes. Apart from this, following this diet plan is beneficial, for brain health, improving cognitive function, and reducing the increased risk of dementia and Alzheimer's disease. Regularly eating a heart-healthy diet along with other physical activities can help in reducing the aging process of the brain and protecting it from several diseases. This kind of eating habit is also known for improving cognitive psychological well-being that can help in improving mental conditions like depression, and stress, and elevates mood.

Apart from this, a Mediterranean diet is focused on whole and fresh foods that aid in healthy, sustainable, and safe weight loss naturally, while it does not promote quick and early weight loss. Consuming fish, animal foods, nuts, and oil helps in effective weight loss when eaten as a significant part of the diet compared to other low-fat vegan foods. Also, eating a Mediterranean diet encourages the intake of oils and nuts which is also beneficial for reducing the risk of type-2 diabetes. However, a Mediterranean eating plan is based upon extracting nutrients from fresh vegetables, fruits, and animal products which neglects the importance of dairy products. Milk and its products are known as the best source of calcium and vitamin D, which are significant for providing nutrition to the bones and keeping the strong and healthy.

DASH Diet

DASH diet stands for 'Dietary Approaches to Stop Hypertension' and is specifically recommended for people who are facing health issues or at risk of developing hypertension or high blood pressure. High blood pressure is a common health issue caused by an inactive lifestyle and inappropriate diet followed by people. Sometimes diabetes and obesity are also responsible for causing hypertension. To combat the negative impacts of high blood pressure, it is mandatory to improve one's living style and switch to a better eating plan, for such reasons, the DASH diet forms one of the best choices to adopt because it flexible and balanced approach and proven heart-healthy results.

DASH diet is focused on consuming food products that have higher quantities of magnesium, calcium, potassium, and fiber. These minerals and substances are known for reducing blood pressure and helping in maintaining healthy blood pressure. Several food items that are rich in the above-mentioned nutrients are fresh vegetables, fruits, lean meat, whole grains, and milk-based products which are low in fat content. While, food items like saturated fats, full-fat dairy products, sweetened beverages, and tropical oils are completely restricted as they are known for increasing blood pressure. The major focus of the DASH diet is to control the intake of food items without restricting the food that is rich in important and beneficial nutrients. This diet plan stress setting guidelines regarding what, when, and how to consume every week to develop a healthy lifestyle. To effectively follow the DASH diet, it is recommended to include fruits, vegetables, complex carbohydrates, lean meats, nuts, seeds, and low-fat dairy products in their diet every day to gain positive results and maintain healthy blood pressure.

Sample Meal Plans

	Day-1	Day-2
Breakfast	• Greek yogurt with walnut or almonds	• Half a cup of instant oatmeal made with low fat milk and one diced banana with one tbsp. peanut butter
Morning Snacks	• One orange	• Sliced pear with cinnamon topping
Lunch	• Three-fourth cup chicken salad, fresh fruit juice, and two whole wheat slices of bread	• Half a cup of roasted beef with one baked potato, and one whole wheat bread
Evening Snacks	• Two plums	• One sliced apple with cinnamon topping
Dinner	• One chicken sandwich made in whole wheat bread and apple juice	• One cup of spaghetti and one cup of mixed green vegetable salad

Health Benefits

DASH diet is a balanced diet plan that restricts the intake of food rich in sodium, fatty milk products, and saturated fats, which helps in reducing the risk of increased blood pressure and several chronic diseases like heart attacks and strokes. Following this type of eating plan on a regular basis could also reduce the risk of obesity and diabetes, and helps to achieve better health. Further, the DASH diet could also help in reducing weight naturally in a sustainable manner as it is focused on eating a diet full of nutrients and completely restricts any food that can cause weight gain. Consistent efforts to follow this diet plan could show positive results without reducing inner strength and causing weakness in the body.

Apart from this, a DASH diet is very easy to follow as it allows consuming several foods with simple recipes and clearly defined delicacies that make it an attractive diet for older adults and young children too. This diet plan emphasizes consuming food rich in fiber, low calories, and having good nutritional values makes it the best choice for feeding growing children. However, the DASH diet has a key feature that stresses reducing the sodium intake from 2300 mg to 1500 mg per day, which can be a complete diet for people who are fit and do not face issues of high blood pressure. Consuming less amount of sodium could gradually increase insulin resistance which can further cause health issues. Further, this diet is a plan not the right choice for people who are suffering from chronic liver and chronic kidney diseases.

Vegan Diet

The specialty of a vegan diet plan is that it is free from any consumption of all types of animal-based products which may be either due to environmental reasons, health benefits, or ethical factors. This eating plan emphasizes consuming only plant-based products that could help in boosting immunity and provide complete nutritional value in a day. Switching to this eating habit would restrict you from consuming meat, poultry, seafood, dairy products, and even honey. Limiting the intake of all kinds of animal-based products excludes all the sources of protein that are derived from them in the form of poultry, fish, eggs, dairy, and meat. However, adopting a vegan diet in a planned and balanced manner could help in supplementing the required protein by consuming plant-based products that are rich in protein. Some of the protein-rich plant-based food products are lentils, peanut butter, tofu, nuts, and red beans. Adopting a vegan diet plan could boost the health benefits with enriched nutrition derived from fresh fruits, vegetables, lentils, whole grains, seeds, and nuts.

Consuming a combination of fruits, nuts, seeds vegetables, lentils, and whole grains, which is the core of every diet plan, helps in acquiring the appropriate requirements of vitamins, minerals, protein, and nutrients that are essential for developing a good and healthy lifestyle.

Sample Meal Plan

	Day-1	Day-2
Breakfast	• One toast topped with peanut butter and sliced banana	• One cup of Greek yogurt sprinkled with blueberries, nuts, and chia seeds
Morning Snacks	• One-fourth cup of dry roasted almonds without salt	• One sliced apple topped with cinnamon
Lunch	• One cup of green vegetable curry with chickpeas and spinach served with half a cup of brown rice	• One Mexican vegetable taco
Evening Snacks	• Hummus with an olive oil topping and green vegetables	• Seven pistachios
Dinner	• Three-fourth cup of green beans curry with half a cup of quinoa	• One cup falafel salad with green vegetables

Health Benefits

Switching to a vegan diet plan from a typical western diet changes the entire eating habits, by eliminating animal-based products and replacing them with only plant-based food products. This emphasizes consuming more amount of a whole-food vegan diet like grains, fruits, vegetables, nuts, seeds, and lentils, which helps in providing higher nutrients to the body. Vegan food products are highly rich in fiber, beneficial plant compounds, several vitamins (like A, C, and E), antioxidants, and minerals like potassium, folate, and magnesium, which help supplement the required nourishment of the body.

Furthermore, hypertension or high blood pressure is one of the major reasons for increasing the risk of several chronic diseases like strokes, heart attacks, and diabetes. However, following a plant-based diet can help in reducing blood pressure which could reduce the risk of these conditions. Apart from this, meat and animal-based products contain saturated fats, which can be bad for our hearts and cause several cardiovascular diseases. Instead, following a plant-based diet can help in consuming food that has anti-inflammatory properties, which is essential for reducing the risk of cardiovascular diseases. Therefore, adding food items like green leafy vegetables, whole grains, nuts, tomatoes, fruits, and extra virgin olive oil can help prevent cardiovascular diseases.

Moreover, a plant-based diet is a healthy and sustainable way to reduce weight naturally, without putting in much effort, which can help in staying healthy and having a good lifestyle. However, a vegan diet restricts the intake of fish and all types of seafood which can cause a deficiency of omega-3 fatty acids that can impact mental health leading to depression. Also, plant-based products can cause a deficiency of vitamin B12 and iron which can increase the risk of anemia. So, it is recommended to follow this diet plan mindfully and in a balanced way, which can help in fulfilling the requirements of calcium, protein, vitamin B12, omega-3 fatty acids, iron, zinc, and iodine.

Chapter 5:

Dos and Don'ts to Eat Well

To keep the body in good health is a duty, otherwise we shall not be able to keep our mind strong and clear. –Buddha, a Spiritual Leader

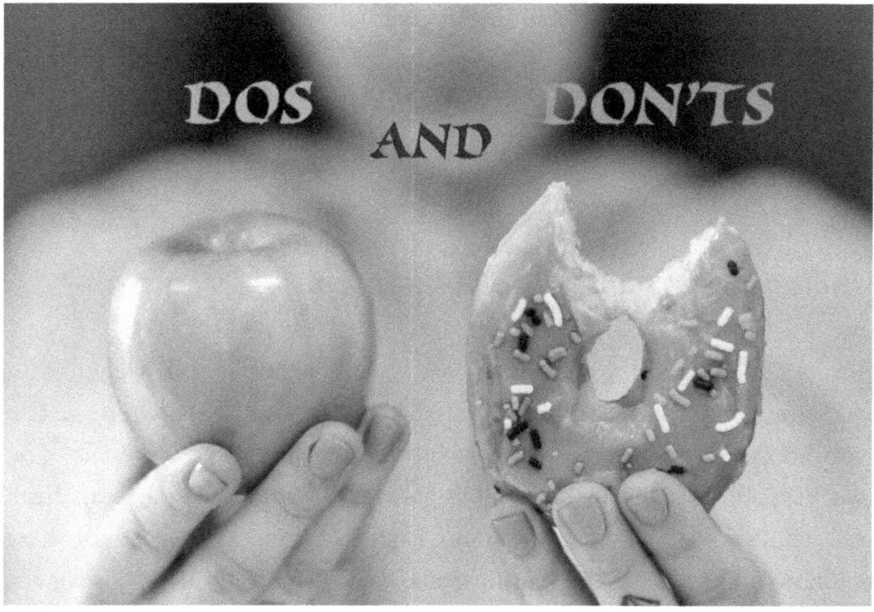

Healthy eating is one of the basic and most important topics that must be talked about. To begin with, there are a variety of diet plans, suggestions about what nutrients are important, and what could be the right definition of healthy food. Healthy food is simply the one that can positively impact our body and boost its overall functioning. While the definition of healthy eating is different for different people. It is because what suits one, may not always be the best for others as well. So, it is important to focus on what type of food and nutrients are most suitable for you, based on your health conditions, appetite, and goals.

Each time when you eat a meal, you are either feeding a disease or fighting against it. The food we consume has immense power to change our life completely, as the food we eat can impact our health conditions. Sometimes, merely the lack of awareness and knowledge about what can be the best healthy eating plan for you is the challenge. However, it is never late to begin this endeavor of eating a healthy diet, as it is simply about being more mindful and conscious of what you are going to eat. So, to make it more clear, more precise, and more effective let's have a look at the common dos and don'ts that will work for all.

Dos For Healthy Eating

Include Fruits and Vegetables in Your Diet

Fruits and vegetables are known for having vitamins, plant chemicals, and minerals that can help in reducing the risk of severe health conditions like digestive issues, blood pressure, heart attacks, and strokes, obesity, etc. It is difficult to gain all the important nutrients from one fruit or vegetable alone. So, it is significant to eat a variety of these which could fulfill all the requirements of vitamins and minerals for the day. Fruits and vegetables are fresh and natural sources of healthy nutrients, which are free from any type of preservatives, artificial colors or sweeteners, and chemical substances. Consuming enough of these foods can help in satisfying the taste buds and also provide several health benefits as they are free from all harmful elements.

Eat in Smaller Portions

It is important to monitor the serving size of the food you eat, which helps in ensuring that you consume a healthy and balanced diet. Eating everything in moderation also helps in preventing overeating, munching excessively on unhealthy foods, or skipping any important nutrient from your meal. Consuming smaller portions of meals at least 4 to 5 times a day can help in losing weight as it improves the metabolism rate. While eating less frequently and larger meals can result in a slower metabolic rate which automatically increases weight. Apart from this eating smaller portion improves the tendency of the body to increase the absorption and utilization of nutrients, efficiently.

A healthy diet must contain a calculative amount of every nutritious food that is required by our body to function properly and maintain good health. Ideally, a portion control diet is more about consuming the average number of calories that are needed by our body to maintain a healthy lifestyle. So, a portioned diet is different for all, as everyone's requirement of daily calories varies from one another. It is better, to keep the size of your dinner smaller than your lunch. While one must ensure that a lunchtime meal must contain green vegetables or salad and also some source of protein like chicken or beef and carbs like whole grains.

Stay Hydrated

Drinking enough water for staying hydrated is one of the most significant aspects of consuming a good diet and maintaining a healthy life. Our body comprises around more than 60% of water. So, staying hydrated can help in keeping the fluid levels in our body topped up, which helps in ensuring that all the functions of the body are performed efficiently. Water is very important for our body, as even a slight reduction in the level of water in our body could make us feel its consequences. Several symptoms like dizziness, dry mouth, lack of concentration, and headaches are common when you are not sufficiently hydrated. Further, poor hydration for longer spans could also lead to constipation, infections in the urinary tract, or even kidney stones.

The daily water requirement for an adult is about 1.5 to 2 liters which can be estimated to be 8 to 10 glasses of water. Intake of water varies from one person to another based upon their level of physical activities and surrounding environment. It is not necessary to wait for the thirst to drink water, as feeling thirsty itself is a sign of dehydration. So, try to drink lots of water as it can help in boosting your physical performance and also improve the functioning of all the vital organs of the body. The best way to identify the symptoms of dehydration is the color of urine. Dark-colored urine is a sign that you are dehydrated and your body needs more water, while a pale-yellow-colored urine indicates a sign of a well-hydrated body.

Follow a Diet Plan

The struggle to eat a healthy diet does not have to be complicated. Adopting a diet plan that helps in gaining all the nutrition required by our body can help in avoiding several health issues. The whole idea of following a strict diet plan is to strive towards developing a healthy life, preventing diseases, maintaining a healthy weight, feeling good about yourself, and gaining complete nutrition. The best way to include all types of healthy food in your meal is to follow a diet plan. Any diet that has proper nutrition must contain enough food that has all the nutritional value and calorie requirements of a day, balanced consumption of solid and liquid foods, and a satisfactory taste to fulfill hunger. However, it's not easy to understand which diet plan would suit you the best, rather it depends upon various factors like height, age, body weight, and physical activities. Apart from this, other important factor is health status and genetic factors. If you have any illness like diabetes, obesity, or malnutrition, or if you have a family history of being obese or diabetic, then you must choose a diet plan based on those factors.

Track Your Meals

Self-monitoring the amount of food that you eat is a positive habit that cannot only help you to track your weight loss but also provides other important benefits. Tracking the meals is a simple way of eating a balanced diet which is the foremost step for developing a healthy lifestyle. Tracking the food you eat is the basis of knowing the number of calories you eat along with evaluating the nutritional content in it. When you track your meals, you are mindful of what you eat and even the size of the meals. It refrains you from unnecessary snacking or skipping meals too. Further, tracking the meals each day also makes you think about your current eating habits. When you are aware of your starting point, it becomes easy and simple to tweak your current eating habit a little bit to attain the nutrition that you need for reaching your goal. By being aware of the daily nutritional and calorie intake you make yourself accountable and conscious of what and why you are eating. While tracking your meals, you must include everything that you eat and drink in a day, portion sizes, and even the time of eating food. Tracking can be made easy with the help of various applications that help in filling in the logs of what you eat and gives a count of your calories and nutritional intake.

Don'ts For Healthy Eating

Avoid Skipping Meals

Sometimes we feel that skipping a meal is the easiest way to reduce weight and maintain a healthy weight. While at times, we skip our lunch and breakfasts to limit the intake of calories for the day. Often, we assume that skipping a meal or two would do no harm to us, and quite obviously it wouldn't starve us to death. However, the consequences of skipping a meal are not good for a healthy life, and could even lead to worsening the situation. Skipping a meal is one of the basic reasons that reduces weight loss and could eventually lead you to gain more weight. Skipping meals slows down the metabolic rate which consequently boosts weight gain. So, skipping meals merely for weight loss is a bad idea.

Apart from this, when you skip meals, your body runs short of blood glucose, which is crucial for the apt functioning of the brain. Lower levels of blood sugar are also responsible for increasing irritable behaviors, fatigue, and confusion, which tends to increase stress and anxiety. It may be difficult to have complete meals at times due to busy days and hectic schedules, so the best way is to have smaller and frequent meals that could provide you with energy for working efficiently the entire day.

Limit Caffeine Intake

Most of us rely on caffeine to jump-start our day which can keep us going to improve concentration and also boost our efficiency to perform our jobs well. However, consuming caffeine beyond the restricted limit can pose serious health problems and is bad for our health. On average around 400 mg of caffeine is the normal intake quantity per day, which equals around 4 cups of brewed coffee. Consuming more than 4 cups of coffee per day can cause several side effects like fast heartbeat, insomnia, headaches, irritability, muscle tremors, nervousness, and frequent urination.

Apart from this, 0.15 tablespoons of pure caffeine powder or 1200 mg of caffeine can be highly toxic as it could even lead to seizures. High doses of caffeine in the form of caffeine powder or any other product can cause serious health issues, including death. So, caffeine despite its qualities of making one feel fresh can have several harmful impacts on human health, if consumed in an uncontrolled way. Thus, cutting down the consumption of caffeine may be unpleasant in the beginning, but with consistency and determination, one can overcome the bad habit of overconsumption of caffeine.

Say No to Added Sugars

Sugar has a sort of bittersweet image in the context of our health. Fresh fruits, vegetables, grains, and dairy products are natural sources of sugar as they are rich in carbohydrates. Consuming these natural sources of sugar is not harmful to our health as it also contains essential minerals, fibers, and vitamins. Our body tends to digest these natural sources of sugar quite slowly, which helps in fulfilling the energy requirements of our body. Apart from this, consuming moderate amounts of fruit and vegetables could also help reduce the risk of several serious diseases like diabetes, cancer, and heart problems.

However, consuming added sugars, either directly, or through other sources like packed fruit juices, beverages, soft drinks, cookies, cakes, flavored yogurts, and candies could have adverse health impacts. Consuming too much-added sugar can increase the risk of several health diseases like diabetes, fatty liver, high blood pressure, weight gain, or inflammation. All these health conditions are dangerous for our heart health as it increases the risk of getting heart attacks or strokes. Therefore, limiting the amount of added sugars is very important to maintain good health by achieving a healthy heart and weight.

Reduce Consumption of Junk Food

Any food that has been canned, pasteurized, frozen, packaged, or cooked is included in the list of processed food. While there are processed foods available in the form of pasteurized milk or dairy products, canned vegetables, and frozen fruits can be included in your healthy diet plan without a second thought. However, consuming any other processed food in the form of cakes, biscuits, rolls pies, chips, sausages, carbonated drinks and many more can prove to be harmful to your health. These highly processed food items contain higher amounts of sugar, salt, preservatives, and additives which can adversely affect your health.

To refrain from eating processed food items you can try to replace them with healthy food of your choice which could provide you with all the necessary nutritional benefits. For instance, substitute unhealthy processed snacking habits with homemade hard-boiled eggs, a variety of nuts, overnight-soaked oats, and some veggies with hummus or fresh fruits. You can drink plenty of water to keep yourself hydrated which could eventually serve more health benefits than carbonated sugary drinks, sports drinks, and sweet tea. Try replacing processed meats like sausages, bacon, lunch meat, and hot dogs with salmon, fresh chicken, or turkey as starters. This entire journey of overcoming bad eating habits with good ones is a time taking process, which needs patience determination, and motivation, so do not rush, take your time.

Refrain from Alcohol

The debate on the health benefits and adverse impacts of alcohol is still hovering over our minds. The only difference that makes alcohol a tonic or a poison is hidden in its dosage. Consuming alcohol more than the moderate limit or getting addicted to it can trigger the risk of life-threatening health issues and disorders. The two-faced characteristics of alcohol must not be a surprise if you booze regularly. Overconsumption of alcohol could have direct and harsh impacts on the functioning of the heart, brain, liver, gall bladder, and stomach. It also affects the cholesterol levels in your blood and causes type-2 diabetes, and cancers. Apart from physical health, alcohol can cause severe harm to your mental health also. Drinking in excess is associated with increased alteration of moods, lack of coordination and concentration, and depression.

Even if you are highly addicted to alcohol consumption, there are better ways to get rid of this bad habit to develop good health and incline yourself towards better things in life. It is very difficult for you completely cut off alcohol consumption overnight, but still, some ways could help you through this struggle. You can set drinking goals for yourself and also maintain notes on dairy that could help you to record the consumption levels. Try to keep yourself busy in outdoor sports, social gatherings, and watching fun movies to avoid thinking about alcohol consumption. Gradually invest in choosing alcohol-free days, which can help you in avoiding these drinks for at least a week or two. Consistency is the key, so keep working towards your goal slowly and steadily until you achieve it, and victory is not far away.

Chapter 6

Perks of Healthy Eating

The food you eat can be either the safest and most powerful form of medicine or the slowest form of poison. —Ann Wigmore, an American Holistic Health Practitioner

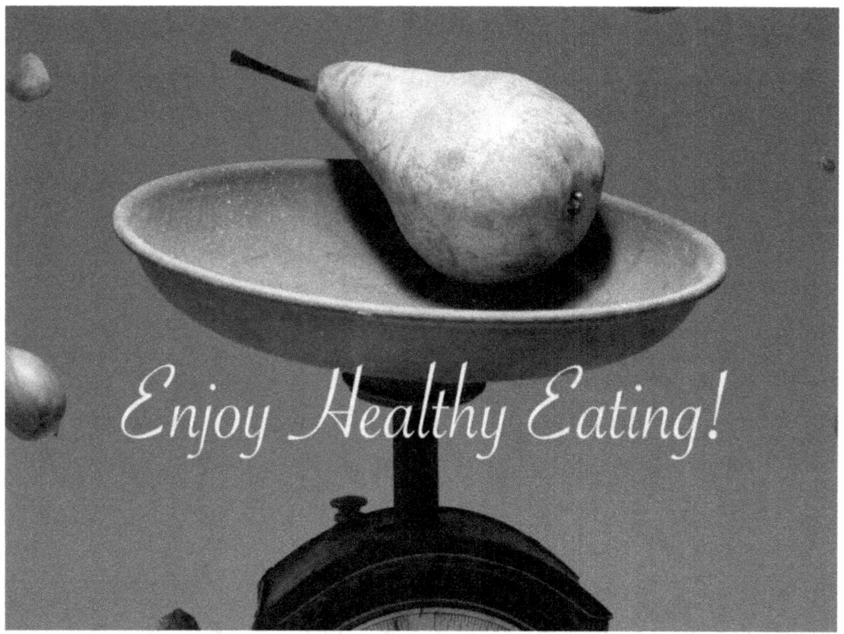

Healthy eating is not a one-size fits all thing, it can be different for different people depending upon their habits, health conditions, lifestyle, and many other minor factors. For those who are underweight and lean, healthy eating may include some more fats, carbs, and loads of proteins, however, it will be entirely different for someone who is obese or overweight. Thus, we cannot set a definition of a healthy diet, instead, we should be mindful of consuming the right quantity of the right food items, that will provide us with the goodness of all the required essential vitamins, minerals, good fats, proteins, and sufficient carbs; for the normal functioning of our body. Moreover, studies have also revealed that taking a balanced diet has proven to be beneficial for us in numerous ways. Our body has a number of vital organs that perform various important tasks for our survival and for the well-being of these organs, we have to nourish our body with the best available food. Hence, to see the positive side of healthy eating, we need to put some effort to improve our eating habits, by following a proper diet and balancing the intake of all the different components of food. So, let's get started with the journey of exploring the perks of eating a healthy diet for our body, mind, and soul.

Boosts Immunity

One of the most unpleasant things in life is falling ill. Although it is not a matter of choice to fall sick or stay healthy, there are some simple and easy tips to keep various illnesses at bay. The best option to fight against various types of health issues is to make your immune system strong enough so that it can fight away any infectious diseases, common flu, viral infections, and other autoimmune diseases with ease. Thus, consuming food items such as various spices, herbs, green leafy vegetables like broccoli, kale, etc., and fruits rich in vitamin C like blueberries, oranges, strawberries, etc., have proven its benefits in boosting the immune system, by providing faster recovery from illnesses and exhibiting quick healing properties. All these healthy food items are a great source of vitamins, minerals, and antioxidants; which are also found in good quantities in several fatty fish, and dairy products like milk, and cheese as well. On the whole, a healthy body with strong immunity can easily fight against any sort of disease and make us fit and energetic.

Improves Heart Health

Our heart is the main functioning unit, as it governs the proper mechanism of all the other organs and helps us feel revitalized by constantly supplying blood to different parts of our body. But, to keep our hearts beating in a good condition, we need to take special care to prevent them from any type of harm. Externally, nature has protected our heart with ribs, but to guard it internally against various diseases, we need to be mindful of our eating habits. Consuming too much salt and unhealthy saturated fats can result in increased levels of cholesterol and high blood pressure issues, which may put our heart at a greater risk of damage. Thus, by maintaining a healthy diet rich in low-fat products, fruits, vegetables, and whole grains; we can reduce the probability of the occurrence of heart diseases. Moreover, including a variety of oily fishes that are a great source of omega-3 fatty acids can work wonders for our heart health. Thus, eating well and avoiding a few unhealthy food items like red meat, alcohol, processed food, etc., can protect our hearts against various illnesses.

Strengthens Teeth and Bones

In the era of glamor and fashion, a beautiful smile is something all of us desire to have, in order to flaunt our mesmerizing personalities. But having a capturing smile cannot be just the magic of your toothpaste, you also need to have a perfect diet that supports healthy teeth as well. A diet that is rich in calcium including all dairy products like milk, cheese, butter, cream, etc., is well suited for enriching our teeth and bones, which prevents the early decay of teeth and bone loss in the form of osteoporosis. Apart from dairy products, calcium can also be obtained from fish like pilchards, salmon, and sardines, green leafy vegetables like broccoli, kale, and other calcium-rich products like legumes, soya, tofu, etc. One very important thing that we must be mindful of while taking calcium is, to make sure we get sufficient vitamin D, either directly from the sun or by eating food loaded with vitamin D like fortified cereals and oily fish, which helps in the absorption of calcium in our body.

Maintains a Healthy Body Weight

Nowadays, people often think that the best way to maintain a healthy body weight is by working out or by exercising regularly. This biggest misconception has diverted the crowd toward gyms and aerobic classes, diminishing the importance of healthy eating and various diet plans that are available. On the contrary, looking at the fact that eating a healthy diet that is rich in fiber like whole grains, fruits, and vegetables, leaves us feeling fuller for a longer time, thereby helping us to cut down any extra intake of calories that are needed to meet the energy demands of the body. Thus, by having a proper diet along with some exercises and workouts, we can maintain a healthy body weight. Moreover, this also helps in reducing the risk of various chronic diseases like diabetes, heart problems, strokes, cancers, etc.; by lowering our cholesterol levels and controlling our blood pressure.

Enhances Digestion

Apart from various vitamins and minerals, dietary fibers and probiotics are the two most important elements that promote proper digestion in our body. Almost all fruits, vegetables, dairy products, and whole grains are rich sources of both probiotics and dietary fibers in our diet. They help our digestive system to work efficiently, by supporting good gut health. Moreover, there are many fermented food items like kefir, miso, buttermilk, and yogurt that contain probiotics, which aid in enhancing our digestion and overall body metabolism. Studies have revealed, that all those following a vegan diet comprising legumes, vegetables, and fruits have regular bowel movements and are less prone to chronic ailments like diverticulitis and bowel cancer. Consuming food that is high in dietary fiber, aids in regulating proper bowel movement, by adding bulk to the stool, which ultimately helps fight constipation.

Reduces Stress

If anyone of you finds it difficult to figure out how eating healthy food can help beat stress, then you must go ahead with this to explore the science behind it. The food we generally eat has a variety of different elements in it, but it is not necessary that any one particular food item will have all the goodness, to maintain a healthy body and mind. Thus, health experts recommend including small portions of many different food items to make a balanced diet. When we take a balanced diet rich in all the vital components of food, our bodies will definitely become fit and we will feel happier and more satisfied.

This sense of contentment that we get from eating a healthy diet, is something that helps in destressing our minds by providing a soothing effect. Moreover, green leafy vegetables and fruits have loads of antioxidants in them, that help in reducing inflammation, thereby easing any sort of physical stress in the body. Eating processed and unhealthy food, that has high levels of sugar and trans fats, gives us nothing other than harming our bodies, as they have no nutritional value. Thus, in a long run, eating light and healthy food can help us in enhancing our mood, by reducing both physical and mental stress, eventually making us feel relaxed.

Increases Life Expectancy

Healthy eating habits directly affect your health and can prove to increase longevity and improve your quality of life. Eating a healthy diet can support decreasing inflammation and reducing the risk of several health disorders like high blood pressure, cancers, heart issues, and diabetes which may improve physical health. Apart from this eating habits can also impact your health span. Healthspan is the maximum time that one feels healthy and nutritious, till the time one needs any sort of medical intervention. Many people surely have longer life spans, but still face many health issues and illnesses for most of their lifetime. Therefore, healthy eating habits are the key to achieving an increased lifespan as well as an improved health span.

Provides Better Sleep

Eating a healthy diet can help in improving the quality of sleep. Several bad habits like eating oily and unhealthy processed food, late-night craving and snacking on junk food items, and irregular dinner timing can impact the smooth biological cycle. Adopting these bad habits as a daily routine can gradually increase the probability of being obese and also cause metabolic syndrome. This could gradually affect digestion, reduce the ability to concentrate, and increase the feeling of uneasiness and discomfort. To combat such negative impacts, it is important to prefer early dinner time at least 3 hours before sleep to improve digestion, reduce stress and provide a sound sleep. Apart from this, other health issues like diabetes, depression, and obesity can also affect the quality of sleep. Therefore, health and sleep are correlated with each other. If you have good health, you will have better sleep and vice versa.

Improves Skin Quality

One of the visible negative impacts of unhealthy eating habits can cause breakouts and acne. Switching your diet from oily and processed food items to healthy and nutritious food can help in achieving healthy skin. A diet that contains fresh fruits, vegetables, seeds, fatty fish, whole grains, and nuts contains nutrients that are beneficial for improving our skin quality. Apart from this drinking lots of water, coconut water, and green tea can also help in giving us glowing and clear skin. One can also try infused water like detox water with citrus fruits and ginger. Apart from this, avoiding refined sugar and trans fats, and maintaining proper hygiene are the secrets that can give you shiny and glowing skin.

Chapter 7:

Obstacles on the Path of Eating Good

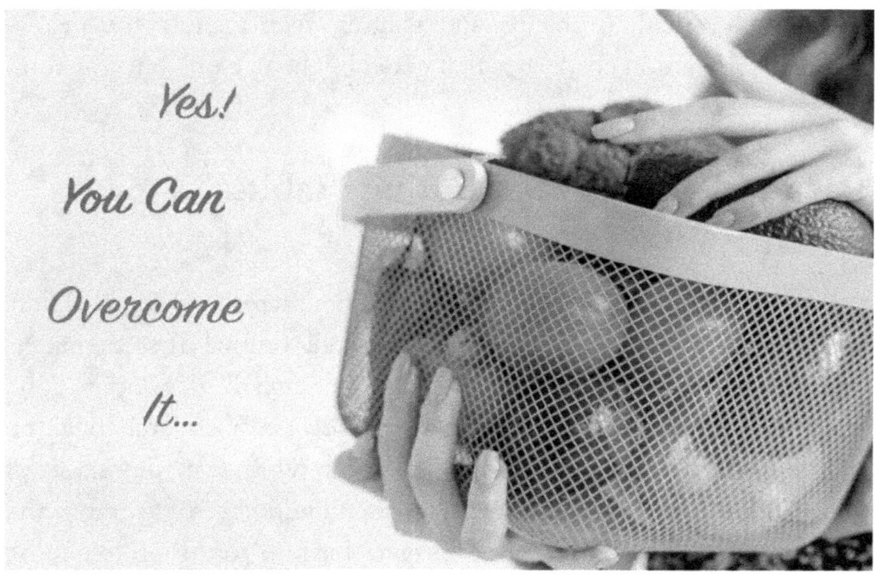

We all are aware of the fact that the quality and portion of food that we
eat has a direct impact on our health. Likewise, every one of us is striving
to achieve a healthy body and mind, as we know what exactly one should
do to accomplish it. Despite the willingness to improve our health and

the knowledge of what to do and how we still find it difficult to achieve good health.

In every sphere of life, we face different challenges, but we always gather hope and courage to look beyond our imperfections and try to move on. Even in this journey of eating healthy and changing our lifestyle, we put in tremendous effort to reach our goal. However, sometimes we may get diverted by various problems, which become big road bumps in the path of our life. Sometimes, lack of time, lower morale, lost willpower, or increased food cravings could hinder the process of eating healthy. Even if you have the best intentions to develop a healthy eating routine, changing your old habits and giving up your addictions is a hard task. So, if you too are on the same road and trying to ditch your unhealthy habits but struggling with problems and failures, then explore the below-mentioned common challenges that could be the one on your way too.

Lack of Time to Plan Eating Habits

One of the biggest struggles that we often come across is the lack of time management to make and plan a healthy eating routine. If something is important to us, we do our best to achieve it. Similarly, developing good health and eating habit is very important, so one must surely buck up and spare some precious time for doing good. While, sometimes, lack of time is the core reason that can create hindrance to learning and exploring a beneficial diet plan. This gives birth to confusion to choose from among the several options and leaves us empty-handed. Therefore, managing time with the correct choice of diet plan is the first step to attaining a healthy eating pattern.

There are many ways to help yourself with beforehand meal and menu preparations. For instance, you can try online groceries shopping, which would help in the easy accessibility of fresh and healthy ingredients to plan your meals. You can also try, jotting down things in a calendar, which could help in providing a clear idea about buying groceries, meal planning for the entire week, and other preparations. Also, keeping a list of quick and easy meals or snacks can help in saving time while you are doing groceries. While, some other useful tricks are to prepare double recipes and freeze the leftovers for later use, or try opting for pre-cut produce to save some time.

Eating Disorders

Eating disorders are psychological conditions of unhealthy eating habits that developed gradually either because of the obsession with body weight, body shape, or any food. Eating disorders are classified as serious mental illnesses which can even be life-threatening if left untreated. These disorders have several symptoms like drastic weight loss, illogical reasons to avoid all meals, patterns of purging and binge eating, consistent denying of the feeling of hunger, extreme fear of weight gain of becoming fat, and many more.

Often, a bad eating habit enters our lives gradually and slowly becomes a permanent part of them. Bad eating habits are like a vicious circle, the more you follow them, the stronger it makes their hold on your lifestyle, leaving dark impressions and sometimes irreparable loss. So, let's discover a few most common and severe eating disorders that can negatively impact our lives.

Binge-Eating Disorder

An eating disorder in which a person eats in an uncontrolled manner until they feel painfully full. This disorder is most common during adolescence or early adulthood, while in some cases it can also be developed later on. A person with a binge eating disorder does not try to restrict calories or adopt purging behaviors like forced vomiting, or excessive exercising to compensate for their binges. The common symptoms of people suffering from this order are eating in secret, overeating, and feeling shame and guilt when reflecting upon the act of binge eating. Anyone suffering from binge eating disorder tends to eat in excess without making a nutritious food choice which may gradually affect their health and may increase the risk of heart attacks, strokes, and type-2 diabetes.

Anorexia Nervosa

Anorexia is one of the most common eating disorders that is generally found in teenagers and young adults, especially in women more than men. In this eating order, the person perceives themselves to be overweight, even if they are underweight. People with anorexia tend to give up healthy eating habits, consistently track their weight, avoid various healthy food items, restrict all their calorie intake, and starve for hours. Anorexia nervosa is categorized into two- restrictive, binge, or purging types. This eating disorder is very dangerous for physical as well as mental health as it can lead to the weakening of bones, thing of hair, brittle nail, and infertility. In severe cases, anorexia can also result in brain, heart, or multiple organ failure which can cause death.

Bulimia Nervosa

Bulimia nervosa is also a well-known eating disorder that is usually common in women as compared to men and is mostly found in teenagers and young adults. In this eating disorder, the person tries to eat unusually larger amounts of food that they don't usually like, for a particular period. Each of these eating episodes continues unless and until the person feels extremely full which may also be painful. The person with a bulimia disorder feels helpless to control or restrict their overeating or binge eating habits which are followed by purging to relieve the discomfort that is being caused. Some of the purging behaviors could be enemas, forced vomiting, fasting, diuretics, and excessive exercise. There are many negative impacts on health because of bulimia disorder like swollen salivary glands, tooth decay, sore throat, hormonal imbalance, severe dehydration, worn tooth enamel, and irritation in the guts. Bulimia can gradually lead to an imbalance in the electrolytes like calcium, sodium, and potassium which could cause heart attacks and strokes.

Pica

Pica is an eating disorder in which the person repeatedly consumes substances that are not regarded as food and also lack any type of nutritional value. This is most common among small children, young adults, and also adults. Anyone suffering from Pica disorder craves eating substances like chalk, soil, dirt, ice, hair, wool, paper, clothes, detergent, laundry, and pebbles. This disorder is common among people who already show signs of intellectual disability, autism spectrum disorder (a developmental issue), and schizophrenia (mental health disorder). People with Pica are more prone to poisoning, undernutrition, gut injuries, and various infections. While in some cases Pica may even cause death depending upon the substance that has been eaten like detergents or other poisonous matter.

Restrictive Food Intake Disorder

Restrictive food disorder was commonly known as 'feeding disorder of infancy and early childhood' and is commonly found among children under the age of 7 years and also in adults. The most common habit in this eating disorder is a disturbed pattern of eating because of various reasons like lack of interest, and dislike of the taste, smell, textures, colors, or temperature of food. The common symptoms of the restrictive disorder are nutritional deficiency, weight loss, lower development in terms of height, lower intake of calories and nutrients, and interference with other social activities like a distraction while eating in public. The restrictive disorder must not be confused with the general picky eating habits of toddlers or reduced eating habits among adults.

Lack of Knowledge

Knowledge is regarded as the prime and foremost tool in the entire process of healthy eating. When we say knowledge, it is not only confined to the understanding of what is good food, and how much is sufficient for a balanced and nutritious diet. Instead, one should also have an awareness of cooking and preparing meals, which is the heart and soul of good eating. Imagine eating a food that does not even tastes, smells, or looks appealing. You will not be able to eat a nutritious diet unless is it prepared in a better manner to make it delicious and worth eating. However, many reasons obstruct the path of gaining knowledge like lack of time, skills, and resources to learn cooking and meal preparations. Well, once you begin exploring, you will find a large variety of online cookbooks, food blogs, Pinterest, and helpful videos which may impart knowledge about clean and hygienic cooking, vegan diet menus, dietary guidelines, favorite cuisines, and food allergies.

Chapter 8:

Threats of Unhealthy Eating

Habits

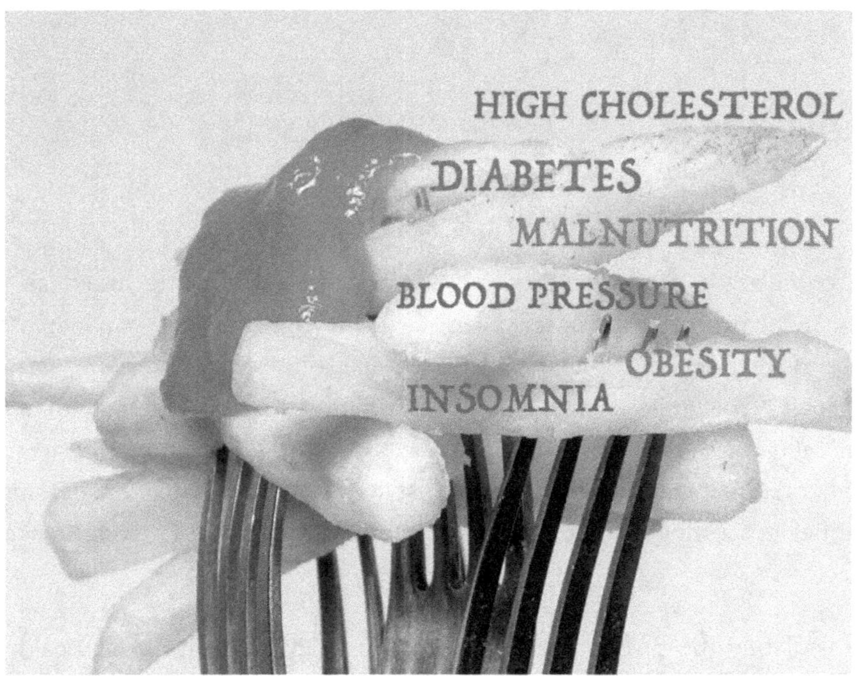

Sometimes, it is not only the determination or lack of inspiration that compels us to eat an unhealthy diet, overeat or eat at the wrong intervals. Instead, it is that bad habit that is developed over time, which we even fail to realize. Leaving home for work skipping breakfast, munching your favorite snack at dinner time while sitting idle in front of the television, focusing only on junkies, or being completely negligent about the food you eat are the common mistakes we make every day unknowingly. But, most of us fail to understand the negative impacts of these adopted bad habits, and how they affect our health and entire lifestyle.

Some health issues are temporary that can be treated with medications, however, the health issues that are caused because of an improper and imbalanced diet cannot be treated with medicines alone. Also, some of these health conditions that occur due to a lack of a nutritious diet can be threatening in some cases and need serious attention at the proper time. So, let's dive deep into this concerning issue and identify the threatening impacts of an unhealthy diet.

Obesity

Obesity is a complex health issue that involves an excessive accumulation of fat in the body. Obesity cannot be regarded as a cosmetic problem, rather it is a serious health condition that can increase the risk of several other health issues like high blood pressure, heart disease, cancers, and diabetes. Several factors are associated with the inability of a person to lose excess body fat. Sometimes, obesity is inherited, a poor and sedentary lifestyle, unhealthy eating habits, and unhealthy eating habits along with environmental and psychological factors.

Calculating the BMI is the best means to analyze if you have a healthy weight based on your height. The body mass index is calculated with your height and weight values. The different range of BMI indicates different weight status which helps in analyzing if you are overweight, underweight, normal, or obese, as shown in the table below:

Body Mass Index (BMI)	Weight Status
Less than 18.5	Underweight
Between 18.5 to 24.9	Normal
Between 25.0 to 29.9	Overweight
More than 30.0	Obese

One of the best ways to get rid of obesity is to reduce some extra body fat and shed weight. Adopting a healthy diet plan, cutting down the extra intake of calories, doing regular work out, and eating at the scheduled time can help in losing weight. Obesity not only impacts physical health but instead it affects mental health too. Obesity gradually deteriorates personal life, as it increases the chances of being discriminated against by others, increasing the chances of social isolation, depression, guilt, shame, hampered self-confidence, and lower achievement at work. Therefore, identifying the threats of obesity at an early stage can help in avoiding the negative consequences on both mental and physical health.

Malnutrition

Malnutrition is a severe health condition that occurs when our body is deprived of the important nutrients, minerals, and vitamins that are essential to maintain healthy organs, tissues, and their functions. Malnutrition develops in two conditions when a person is undernourished or over-nourished. Malnutrition has affected people globally, especially because of their lifestyles, eating habits, environment, and available resources. To prevent the health condition of malnutrition, one must put efforts into following a diet plan that could help in alleviating the root cause of overnutrition or undernutrition in our body. A balanced diet to prevent the occurrence of malnutrition must include a variety of foods like carbohydrates, fats, protein, minerals, vitamins, and water.

Undernutrition

Undernutrition happens when the food and nutrients you consume are excreted more frequently than compared to the normal rate at which they are consumed and absorbed. Another major reason for undernutrition is eating an imbalanced diet that has lower nutrient content. Eating a balanced and portioned diet is the key to overcoming the signs of undernutrition. Those suffering from severe undernutrition must consume food supplements, zinc, and iron or iodine pills or must consult a health care professional in severe cases.

Overnutrition

Overnutrition is caused when you eat too much, follow an imbalanced diet, eat at the wrong time, eat an unhealthy diet like excess of processed foods, follow an inactive lifestyle, or consume several supplements of vitamins or other nutrients. Further, with the changing dietary habits of consuming food with high fat and salt, the risk of being overweight is increasing rapidly which may also increase blood pressure. Consuming healthy food that involves lots of fresh fruits, vegetables, grains and lentils, healthy oil and fats, seeds, and nuts along with vigorous physical activities can help in getting rid of nutrition which could reduce the chances of obesity, overweight, and high blood pressure.

High Cholesterol

Cholesterol is a wax-like substance that is present in the blood to build and keep the cells healthy. However, higher content of cholesterol in the blood could increase the deposits of fats in the blood vessels. Gradually with time, these excessive fat deposits tend to block the way for easy flow of blood through the arteries. In severe conditions, these blockages due to fat deposits can form a clot increasing the chances of heart attacks and strokes. So, higher levels of cholesterol in the blood can result in dangerous conditions and increase the risk of severe heart diseases.

Sometimes, the condition of high cholesterol is inherited, while the most common cause is the intake of unhealthy food that results in increased blood cholesterol levels. There are two types of cholesterols, low-density lipoprotein (LDL) and high-density Lipoprotein (HDL). LDL is the bad cholesterol that gradually tends to accumulate in the walls of arteries, causing blockage and inefficiency of the blood vessels to carry the blood. While HDL is the good cholesterol that functions as picking up the excess cholesterol and back to the liver. To prevent the high cholesterol condition, one must choose a diet that is free from all types of saturated and Trans fats, which are known for increasing the LDL cholesterol.

Instead, consume a diet with low salt content, rich in fruits, whole grains, and vegetables. Avoid consuming any source of animal fats, instead replace them with good fats that too in moderation. Keep away from any bad habits like smoking, drinking, and quite a sedentary lifestyle. Doing regular workouts and having an active lifestyle are important factors that can help in avoiding the consequences of high cholesterol.

Fluctuating Blood Pressure

Fluctuations in blood pressure may occur due to performing vigorous physical activities, while in some cases this fluctuation can also signal any serious health issue. With a small fluctuation the blood pressure, our body would not show any signs and symptoms. However, in conditions where the blood pressure rises too much above the normal range or reduces too low, your body will show certain symptoms. The ideal blood pressure range for a healthy adult is 120/80 mm Hg or slightly less than that. Any rise in blood pressure above this range could show the symptoms of headaches, bleeding from the nose, or shortness of breath. If left untreated, high blood pressure can increase the risk of strokes, heart attacks, and various other serious health conditions.

Apart from this, any reading of blood pressure less than 90/60 mm Hg is regarded as low blood pressure. Most often, low blood pressure has no severe signs and symptoms, however, it can cause fainting and dizziness in some people. Low blood pressure is not a sign of good health, as a very low reading could be life-threatening. There are several causes of low blood pressure dehydration, any heart-related condition or disease, pregnancy, allergic reactions, infection, and improper intake of diet.

Any fluctuation in blood pressure below or above the normal range can cause serious problems. The best way to avoid such complications other than medications is to adopt a healthy lifestyle. The food we consume is one of the basic reasons that can affect the blood pressure in our body. To control high blood pressure, you must adopt a DASH diet plan which focuses on eating low-dairy products, whole grains, vegetables, and fruits. Reduce the intake of sodium, alcohol, tobacco, and caffeine products. You must also invest time in losing extra weight and improve your physical activities through regular exercise. Apart from this, to prevent the symptoms of low blood pressure, focus on eating smaller portions of a meal with a strict routine of low carb diet plan. Drinking lots of water can helps in preventing dehydration while avoiding alcohol and caffeine. Doing regular workouts could also help in improving this health condition.

Various Diseases

Developing a healthy lifestyle is the secret behind feeling good, while it can also serve the benefits of keeping you far away from several preventable diseases and health conditions. Gaining an appropriate amount of nutrition is fundamental for living a healthy life. Poor and inadequate nutrition is the consequence of poor eating habits, or not consuming enough and a complete diet. The failure to choose a balanced diet that fulfills all the requirements of nutritious food may lead to several health conditions like increased risk of diabetes, anemia, rickets, heart-related diseases, osteoporosis, and several types of cancers.

Apart from this, the deficiencies of various nutrients can cause scurvy, hypoglycemia, beriberi, pellagra, etc. Deficiency or over intake of nutrients can disrupt the functions of the body like altered metabolism rate, bone formation, immune function, muscle formation, and cognitive functions. Therefore, it is important to consume a healthy diet with a conscious mind to include all the nutrients in the diet that can help in meeting the basic requirements of our body.

Digestive Issues

Most digestive problems are related to the food you eat and other diet-related factors. Eating a lot of processed food, sugar, and beverages, while avoiding fresh fruits, vegetables, and fiber can affect the function of your digestive system. Eating an inadequate amount of nutrients can cause an imbalance in the production of necessary enzymes that support digestion. Some of the most common digestive issues like constipation, gallstones, diverticular diseases, etc., are highlighted below:

Constipation

Eating a fiber-rich diet reduces the risk of constipation which helps in saving time and discomfort. Constipation can make you feel bloated, increased straining, slow bowel movement, and difficulty to eliminate dry and hard stool. Constipation is a temporary condition that can be improved by eating fiber-rich foods that help in moving stool through the digestive tract and easing discomfort.

Gallstones

A diet that has a higher intake of fats and cholesterol but a lower intake of fiber can increase the risk of getting gallstones. Gallstones are solid substances that are made up of bile and get accumulated in the gall bladder. Bile is secreted in the liver and contains protein, bile salts, bilirubin, cholesterol, and water. Bile is stored in the gall bladder and is released when our body needs to break down fats. Getting gallstones is a severe health condition, that shows symptoms like nausea, pain in the right side of the upper abdomen, fever, and greyish stools. This condition can be life-threatening if no serious action is taken on time.

Diverticular Diseases

Constipation is the root cause of diverticular disease. Diverticula are protruding pocket-like extensions that are formed from the colon. Due to increased problems of constipation and using force for eliminating hard stools, these small pouches are formed. If it is left untreated, these pouches can get infected which results in diverticulitis and inflammation of that area. The common symptoms include pain in the left abdomen diarrhea, nausea, bloody stools, constipation, vomiting, and fever.

Sleep Disorders

Nowadays, aiming for getting a night of sound sleep is one of the most overlooked issues, as we are so occupied with our daily activities, that we don't spare some quality time to take rest and relax. On top of that our unhealthy eating habits serve as icing on the cake, by curbing any possibility to soothe and calm our minds and body. Although it is not a difficult task to understand that our sleeping routine and eating habits are closely interrelated and have a complex relationship between them, we don't bother to make a change.

Studies have revealed that there are various components in food items that can disrupt the normal sleeping pattern, either by shortening or lengthening one's sleep cycle. It is recommended to focus on a diet rich in vitamins and minerals, as they are important for the normal functioning of our vital organs, thereby promoting stress-free sleeping time. Apart from this, there are various serious disorders that are triggered due to unhealthy eating habits like obstructive sleep apnea (OSA), nocturnal eating syndrome (NES), etc., which leave a negative impact on both the physical and mental well-being of an individual. Thus, it is necessary to understand the importance of mindful eating which can eventually optimize our sleep patterns and guide us toward a healthier lifestyle.

Poor Efficiency

Comparing the current modern ways of eating to that of the old traditional ways can probably give us goosebumps, as it will help us see and understand the drastic change in the nutritional value of the food, that has come over the ages. Various research in this field has been conducted, to study the impact of eating different types of food items on longevity, health, and overall efficiency of an individual. Nowadays, the consumption of processed food has increased a lot, due to several reasons like lack of time, busy work life, lack of awareness, etc., which has ultimately disturbed the balance in our bodies.

This unhealthy way of eating is working as a slow poison for us, by damaging our internal organs and disrupting their normal functioning. All this eventually results in various health problems like heart diseases, strokes, diabetes, obesity, etc., due to the absence of essential nutrients that are necessary for our survival. Moreover, these health conditions result in low energy levels, lethargy, and restlessness, thereby influencing the quality of performance of an individual both on professional and personal fronts. Hence, including an unhealthy diet in our lifestyle, can lead to low efficiency which will have a negative impact on mental well-being as well, pushing one toward stress, depression, and gloominess.

Chapter 9: Myths About Healthy Eating

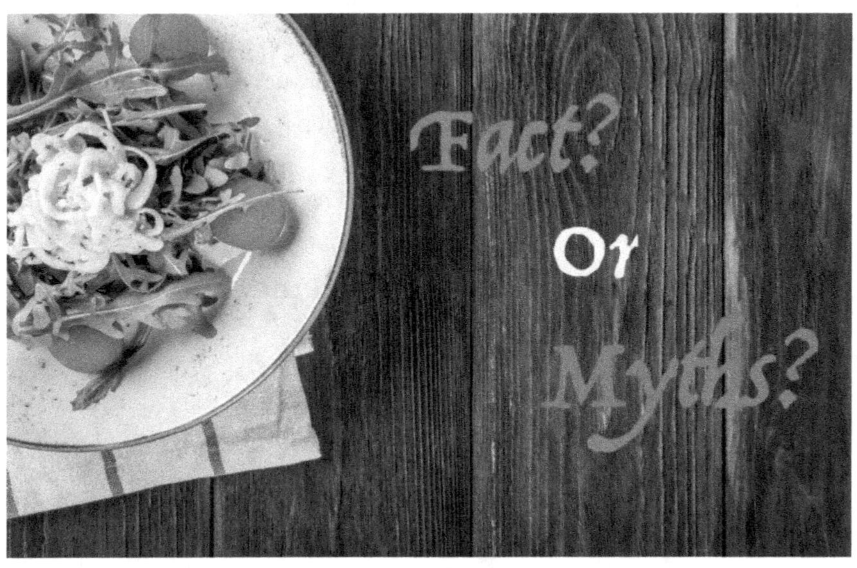

Advancements in science and technology has not only helped to make our lives easier and simpler but, have also improved our sense of understanding, as gaining information about anything is not a challenging task anymore. Nowadays, all the facts that we want to explore about our lives, diet, eating habits, and healthy living are just a click away. However, just scrolling down social media posts, several web pages, and other interactive groups does not necessarily impart correct knowledge about everything we want to explore.

Similarly, when you are enthusiastic about investing in a healthy lifestyle, endless questions may hover in your mind and the only option we have is to explore the answers ourselves. Alas, sometimes putting in these efforts could end up creating new problems or dilemmas for us. So many people, so many talks, and so many myths, which stand true even in the case of eating healthy. We are often lost and confused, as to what to follow and what not. Thus, choosing a diet that could improve our health or deteriorate it, completely depends on our trust and faith in ourselves and the food we eat. The only way to help ourselves make the correct choice and adopt healthy eating habits is, to gather in-depth information about the rising issue. So, let's discuss and explore several myths associated with healthy eating habits, which often restrict us from following the right path.

Eating Carb-Rich Food is Unhealthy

Carbohydrates are one of the most important nutrients that helps in providing energy to our entire body to function properly and efficiently. Not all carbs are bad, instead, the carbs that are derived from fresh fruits, vegetables, whole grains, nuts, and dairy play an important role to boost your health. However, the carbs that are obtained from sources like refined sugar and refined grains in the form of baked cookies, cakes, sweetened beverages, and white bread are not considered to be healthy and must be avoided.

A Vegan Diet is a Healthier Option

It's easy for us to imagine ourselves losing extra kilos and achieving a healthy body only by switching to a vegan diet plan. However, staying healthy is not about choosing a vegan diet, rather it is more about eating the food that is healthy for you. If you simply rely upon a vegan diet and eat lots of fried foods like vegetable nuggets and French fries, it would do no benefit to you. Infect, such type of unhealthy vegan food could instead deteriorate your health further. Avoiding meat, poultry, and fish from your diet could create an imbalance in the nutritional value. So, you must be mindful while selecting the vegan meal plan to ensure that it has different types and sources of nutrients available to make your diet a perfect layout for achieving good health.

Eating Fruits Increases Blood Sugar

Consuming fruits can help in reducing the risk of various diseases like high blood pressure, obesity, heart diseases, cancers, and heart strokes. If you are suffering from diabetes then it is important to consume fruits as it can prevent the occurrence of the above health conditions. Fruits are a rich source of several important vitamins, minerals, and soluble and insoluble fiber which improves bowel movement and improves health. To manage diabetes, it is important to manage blood fats, blood pressure, long-term blood glucose levels, and weight. Eating fruits can play a positive role in managing the above conditions. The glycemic index of most fruits is low to medium which does not lead to any sharp hike in the blood sugar level. However, portion size is an important factor that must not be ignored while consuming fruits. Eating fruits in moderation or in small slices would not be harmful while eating larger portions of fruits is not healthy for people suffering from diabetes.

Eating Fatty Foods Will Make You Fat

Most of us are scared to try fatty foods, as it may increase our weight. Fat is an important nutrient that helps in absorbing various fat-soluble micronutrients like vitamins A, D, and E. Without sufficient fats in our body these core nutrients could not get absorbed in our body and may affect our health. Eating fats in the form of plant-based products like nuts, seeds and avocados and olive oil are the best sources of fats that help in the proper functioning of our body and also maintain our weight. Eating fats is not bad, but controlling portion size is the key to extracting the best benefits from healthy sources of fats.

Calories are Always Unhealthy

Calories are the basic unit to count the energy, that is required for maintaining our healthy living. We cannot survive without sufficient calorie intake, as it acts like the currency for the powerhouse of energy in our body, which assists in the normal functioning of all the different organs. Sometimes, in some medical conditions or diets, the intake of calories can be minimized by employing different ways. Thus, choosing the right source of calories can make the difference that we are looking for. So, instead of eliminating calories completely or reducing the levels of calorie intake, we should go ahead with a feasible diet plan that meets the required calories in a balanced manner. Moreover, consuming a low-calorie diet can help in reducing weight initially, but when considering long-term goals, it is not a viable choice. Continuing a low-calorie diet, below 1200 calories per day can gradually affect our metabolism rate and in turn, slows down the burning of extra calories which could restrict further weight loss.

Eat Breakfast Like a King

We all have grown up listening to a very old saying that breakfast must be consumed like a king, as it is the prime meal of the day that provides nutrition and energy to keep us active the entire day. While, this is not true in every case, especially for adults, as skipping breakfast can help them in reducing the intake of excess calories at the start of the day. Moreover, during intermittent fasting which helps in quick and efficient weight loss, breakfast is usually skipped or taken in the later part of the day. This has proved to serve endless health benefits, which include a reduction in inflammatory markers and controlled blood sugar levels. However, skipping breakfast is not recommended for growing children, teenagers, and pregnant ladies, as they need timely nutrition to maintain their good health and a proper growth rate.

Chapter 10:

Get Inspired to Eat Well

To eat is a necessity, but to eat intelligently is an art. –La Rochefoucauld, a
French Author

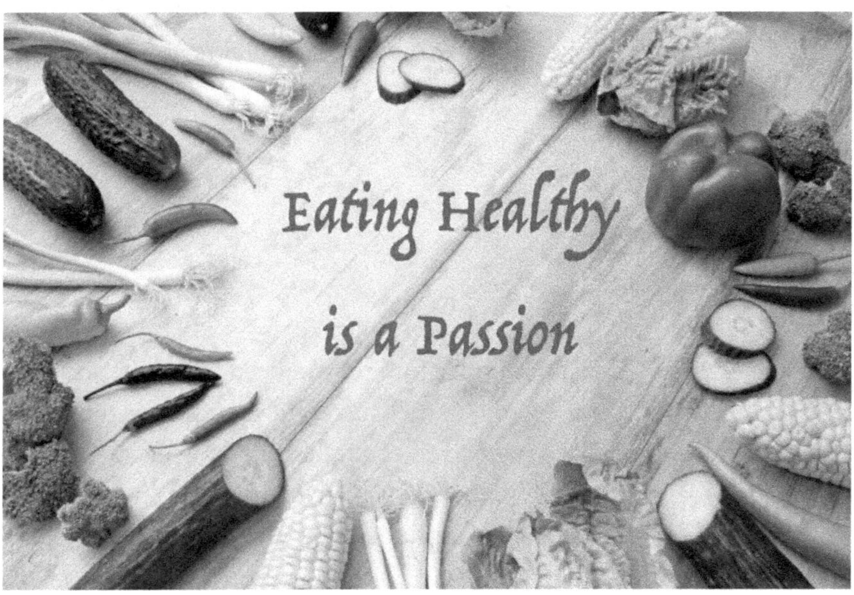

Sometimes, in the journey of life, when you feel sluggish, exhausted, and
ready to give up, just then even a small ray of hope can work wonders
by motivating us through our tough times. This motivation to keep going
on ahead is something we often acquire from our famous star celebrities
or eminent personalities, whom we all look up to as role models. The
actions of these great men and women undoubtedly inspire us for many
reasons and give us immense hope and courage to strive for what we are
looking for in our lives. In the glamor and shine of this world, the
endeavor to achieve good health is a demanding task as it compels us to

give up all our bad habits, addictions, and a sedentary lifestyle, which is a must for staying fit and healthy.

At times, we get tired of fighting against all the negativities around us, but then as we look at the ideal lives of these celebs, it acts as a powerful and driving force that pushes us toward aspiration and desires to look and live like them. Thus, it helps us to look at our lives differently, adopt new ideas, and follow the encouraging footsteps of our role models, to bring about a positive change in ourselves and our lifestyles. So, let's discover the hidden secrets of a few of the most influential public figures who have left no stone unturned to steer their fitness revolution all over the world.

Brad Pitt

If you follow a diet that makes you feel healthy both physically and mentally, then age is just a number for you. Brad Pitt, an American star icon who serves as a strong role model and an inspiration for the young generation, has successfully achieved the milestones of staying healthy. The secret behind Brad Pitt's healthy lifestyle is hidden in his simple seven meals plan per day, which includes some kind of lean protein in each of his meals. Further, to balance this type of diet, the actor invests in regular and intensive workouts for six days a week, out of which two days are specifically dedicated to cardio training. Thus, his relentless determination, healthy diet plan, and highly active lifestyle are the biggest secrets of Brad Pitt's unbeatable fitness. Brad Pitt is a great example for all his fans out there, who strive for a fitter body and a healthier lifestyle, to accomplish their goals with strong willpower and dedication.

Jennifer Aniston

Most of the time, the diet plans of famous personalities are considered to be restrictive, which makes it a difficult choice for any normal person to follow them. However, the famous American actress, Jennifer Aniston who is well known for her acting skills and stunning beauty, has a fixed diet plan that is quite handy for anyone out there. Jennifer Aniston follows a wholesome diet, avoiding the consumption of sugar and processed food, which helps her maintain her glowing skin and perfect health both physically and mentally. Apart from this, she is a long-term yoga enthusiast, which assists her to keep a balance between her mind, body, and soul.

Chloe Burrows

Chloe Burrows, a 25-year-old rising social media influencer, who has already achieved enough fame and appreciation through her professional and personal accomplishments, is a role model for all her followers. Being a fitness fanatic, Chloe Burrows follows a balanced diet plan with special emphasis on protein smoothies. These protein smoothies are included in her everyday morning routine, to charge her up for hitting the gym. Apart from this, she keeps herself hydrated by drinking around 2 ½ liters of water per day with a squeeze of any citrus fruit like orange, tangerine, lemon, or grapefruit, enhancing the taste of water with its natural sweetness. Staying hydrated, having protein smoothies, and working out in the gym regularly, are a few simple yet effective healthy life hacks that have helped Chloe Burrows to achieve glowing clear skin, a healthy body, and mental soundness.

Lucy Liu

Lucy Liu, a rising American actress who is a pure vegetarian, firmly believes that eating healthy food is the heart and soul of accomplishing healthy living. Being a vegetarian for the last five years, Lucy Liu follows a strict vegan diet that could help her gain all the necessary nutrients and benefits from plant-based products alone. Lucy Liu prefers to go with organic sources of food because she is concerned about achieving good health without disturbing nature. Apart from the balanced diet plan, she also extracts her daily dose of vitamins and minerals through multivitamin pills, which help her to develop a stronger immune system and fight away any type of illnesses. Moreover, she invests some of her precious time in working out, to keep herself physically active and fit along with doing some Pilates to keep her body in good shape.

Tom Cruise

In today's dynamic world, maintaining a balance between our work life and personal life is the biggest challenge, which often diverts our attention from doing anything good for our health and fitness. Tom Cruise, a highly dedicated and award-winning global star is leading us by example, in how he maintains a balance between his personal and professional priorities. He follows a simple low-carb diet that is restricted to 1200 calories per day and completely avoids any processed or oily foods. Tom Cruise, relies more on healthy snacking in the form of fresh fruits and nuts. He prefers meals with grilled meat, chicken, and fresh vegetables. Apart from a healthy eating plan, Tom Cruise consciously invests in gym workouts like cardio and weight training exercises to improve his body metabolism, muscle endurance, ripped abs, and muscular physique. Moreover, the star maintains a physically active lifestyle, with his enthusiasm for outdoor sports activities like running, hiking, kayaking, etc., which helps him achieve a healthy body, mind, and soul along with his fun-filled adventures.

Kate Hudson

All those who are very much fitness conscious, may be aware of the name Kate Hudson, who is a health and wellness freak and leaves no chance to inspire others with her incredible lifestyle. The lady star who is famous for being in shape even at this age is highly conscious about what she eats in a day which makes her energetic, glowing, and sculpted. Kate Hudson believes in following a portioned diet, which is basically divided into five small portions for the day. Her healthy diet is comprised of a list of food item that helps her achieve complete and balanced nutrition through lean protein, whole grains, plant-based foods, healthy fats, loads of fresh fruits, and nuts. However, she completely avoids food items like processed meat, refined sugar, unhealthy fats, caffeine, gluten, and dairy products. Apart from this, walking, working out, and doing Pilates are her everyday routine, which helps her to burn out extra calories and maintain the balance between her mind and body.

Chapter 11:

Interesting Facts About Healthy Eating

Your diet is a bank account. Good food choices are good investments. –Bethenny Frankel, an Entrepreneur

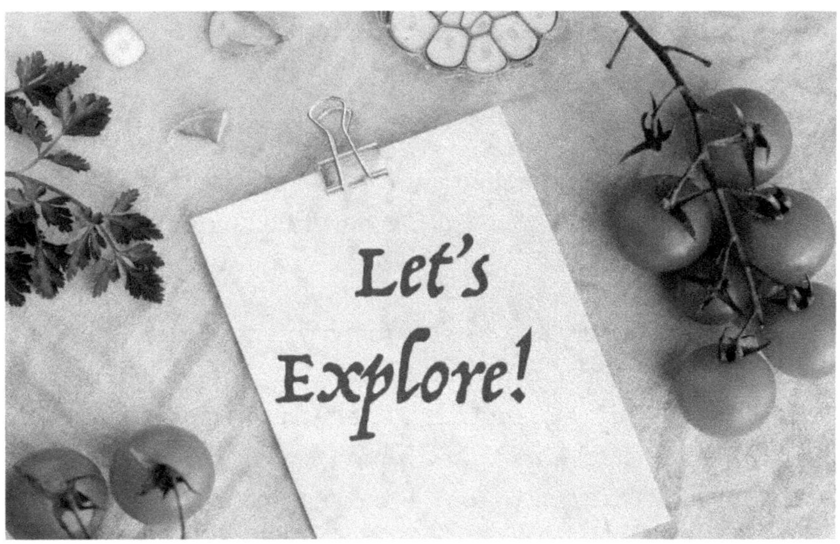

After exploring a whole lot of new things about food and learning unique and simpler ways to maintain good and healthy eating habits, it's time to

have some fun with a few interesting and helpful facts that may surely leave you astonished:

1. All people are unique and no diet is a perfect fit for all, one needs to do little experiments to figure out the best diet plan for oneself.

2. One should include a lot of seasonal fruits and veggies in their daily diet, as they are a great source of nutrition and can help one stay healthy.

3. Consuming junk food has become the root cause of most chronic health disorders like heart disease, obesity, blood pressure fluctuation, etc., which can be fatal.

4. Fruits and vegetables are rich in water and fiber which form roughage in our digestive system and help ease bowel movement, thereby preventing constipation.

5. Eating food items rich in vitamin B4 like yogurt, eggs, legumes, and nuts can help one get a night of uninterrupted and sound sleep.

6. There are a number of spices that have extraordinary medicinal properties and are used worldwide to cure various types of illnesses and health problems. For instance, cardamoms are used to ease digestive issues, cinnamon has antioxidant properties, carrom seeds are used to relieve cough and cold, etc.

7. Honey can preferably be used as a replacement for white sugar like in baking recipes, tea, lemonade, etc.

8. Drinking fresh juice is a better choice than having processed drinks as the former are rich in essential nutrients necessary for staying fit and healthy.

9. Green leafy vegetables like chards, kale, rockets, etc., are considered superfoods, as they are a great source of phytonutrients, vitamins, and minerals that slow the aging process.

10. The best way to fight depression and sleep disorders is to consume a small quantity of nutmeg powder mixed in milk, just before bedtime, as it has a calming effect on the mind.

11. Refined sugar that has loads of calories can be alternatively replaced by natural sweeteners like stevia, yacon syrup, monk fruit, etc., that contain a negligible amount of calories and can be an awesome tastemaker for those suffering from diabetes.

12. All colorful vegetables like carrots, beetroot, tomatoes, broccoli, etc., are rich in beta-carotene, which is vital for maintaining healthy skin.

13. When going for frozen or tinned food items, one should always check the ingredients and opt for a low-sugar and salt product, as processed foods contain extra added sugar and salt to preserve food for a longer time.

14. Experts suggest that one should plan each of their meals by focusing on starchy food items like pasta, wholegrain cereal, whole meal bread, etc., as they are energy-providing food and will keep one charged for a longer time without making one feel empty on their stomach.

15. While opting for cheese, one should go ahead with some strongly flavored cheese like cheddar, as you can enjoy its intense taste even in smaller portions which will help one cut down some fats.

16. When one thinks of consuming fish, it is best to have it in a baked, steamed, or grilled form rather than frying it, as it enhances its flavors and makes it a healthier choice.

17. Although all fats are loaded with calories, there are some healthier fats too which are known as good unsaturated fats and help lower the risk of various diseases.

18. We must keep ourselves hydrated by consuming approximately 2-3 liters of water a day, accompanied by various water-rich fruits and vegetables that can add to the body's fluid.

19. Most plant-based oils like olive oil, rapeseed oil, etc. are rich in unsaturated fats, which can assist in lowering cholesterol, thereby reducing the risk of heart problems and blood pressure issues.

20. Butter can be replaced by any low-fat unsaturated oil like olive oils, flaxseed oils, etc., as they are a healthier choice.

21. Onions are best when used in a raw or slightly cooked form, as they are a rich source of antioxidants and detoxify our body. Hence, overcooking onions deprives one of their beneficial anti-histamine, anti-allergy, and anti-viral properties.

22. Broccoli is a super veggie, as it contains the goodness of calcium as in whole milk and has twice as much vitamin C as in orange.

23. It is best to have green underripe bananas as they are a good source of prebiotics and have low sugar content compared to over-ripped bananas. However, yellow over-ripped bananas are rich in potassium, and vitamin B6 which help to maintain normal blood pressure.

24. Using Fresh chili peppers in food not only enhances the flavors of the food but also helps to burn extra calories.

25. Those who love to eat chocolates as a mood elevator can easily replace them with roasted cocoa bean powder without adding sugar to boost themselves.

26. Dates when taken empty stomach serve as the best source of iron and help in fighting against anemia.

27. One should prefer white meat over red meat, as the latter is not too good for health reasons and increases the risk of strokes, cancers, heart diseases, and diabetes.

28. Apart from meat, lentils are the best vegan source of protein and assist in maintaining the overall health of an individual.

29. Eating fruits and vegetables regularly results in healthy glowing skin as they are a rich source of vitamins and minerals.

30. Healthy omega-3 fatty acids are not produced by our body, hence the best way to consume them is to feast on seafood which helps to maintain strong, healthy, and shiny hair.

31. It is okay to consume some more calories occasionally, as you can always burn the extra ones by working out or maintaining an active lifestyle.

32. Researchers have revealed the recommended calorie intake of women which is about 2000 calories a day, which differs from the basic requirement of men which is approximately 2500 calories per day.

33. It is recommended that one should consume at least 5 different varieties of fruits and vegetables every day, to see a noticeable difference in their health and body's metabolism.

34. One should mindfully cut down the intake of sugary food and drinks, as it can lead to tooth decay and obesity.

35. Experts suggest that one should avoid skipping one's breakfast, as it is the most important meal of the day. The best way to plan

your breakfast is to arrange a low-sugar, high-fiber, and oil-free meal that would work wonders to stay fit and healthy.

36. Including edible seeds like pumpkin seeds, flaxseeds, chia seeds, etc., in your diet is a good way to add loads of essential vitamins and minerals that can provide energy and boost your immune system.

37. Although nuts like almonds, peanuts, walnuts, cashews, etc., are high in calories, they can be used as one's favorite snack as they have healthy unsaturated fats that help in digestion and makes you feel full for a longer time. But, be mindful to eat these nuts in moderation to prevent excess calorie intake.

38. Frozen yogurt is a great substitute for ice creams, as the former is low in calories and contains probiotics that can be gut-friendly and a good source of calcium as well.

39. Milk has an impressive nutritional profile and a glass of milk is packed with a broad array of vitamins, minerals, proteins, antioxidants, and healthy fats that helps to maintain strong and healthy teeth and bones.

40. For those suffering from lactose intolerance, non-dairy milk like soy milk, almond milk, hemp milk, rice milk, etc., are the best alternative to replace dairy milk.

41. Research has confirmed the fact that eating slowly is a good habit, as it gives time for your brain to perceive the signals that whether you are full or hungry and this helps in reducing the calorie intake, thereby controlling your weight.

42. Although Greek yogurt is higher in fat and protein than regular yogurt, it is a good choice for those who aim to opt for a low-carb diet and have lactose intolerance.

43. Having eggs for breakfast is a healthier alternative, as it keeps you full for a longer period of time and helps you consume fewer calories while having other meals like lunch and dinner.

44. Drinking a glass of warm lemon water about 10-15 minutes after the meal can surely help you fight the issues of bloating, heartburn, and constipation by speeding up the process of digestion and is also helpful in losing some extra kilos.

45. One of the best ways to replenish your body with water and to stay hydrated is by consuming water-rich fruits and vegetables like watermelon, musk melon, cucumber, oranges, peaches, strawberries, etc., that helps fight various health problems like kidney stones, urinary tract infections, and even kidney failure.

46. Olives are rich in antioxidants and oleic acids, which make them beneficial to fight against cancer and bone loss.

47. Using too much salt in your meal may raise your sodium level, resulting in high blood pressure which triggers heart problems. Thus, salt should be consumed in moderation to maintain your overall health.

48. Apple cider vinegar can work wonders for those who are obese as it renders a feeling of fullness that naturally cuts off your calorie intake, thus helping in shedding weight easily and being healthy.

49. While having fish, one should be mindful that many fishes like sharks, swordfish, gemfish, barramundi, etc., have a high content of mercury in them which can be highly poisonous if consumed in large quantities.

50. For maintaining good eye health, one should consume food items that are rich in vitamin A such as carrots, mangoes, papaya, fish, eggs, dairy products, etc.

Conclusion

"Eating Well for a Healthy Lifestyle" is an inspiring book for all of you who wish to stay fit and smart, using the miraculous power of eating good and healthy food. This book is a journey of life, that will teach you simple and easy ways to maintain your health by learning and exploring various unveiled aspects of eating a healthy diet. The book provides you with a wonderful guide, to the different food items that are available and their sources, so that you can easily decide whether to opt for a vegan or a non-vegan diet pattern. Apart from that, the book highlights the basic components of food i.e, proteins, fats, carbs, vitamins, minerals, fiber, and water, that are vital for the normal growth and development of our mind and body. Moreover, this book is the best guide for all those who are struggling to decide on a specific diet plan, as it covers almost all the trending diet plans that are recommended by dietitians.

This book is a true gem for all those who are fitness freaks and aim to change their lives by simply making a few changes in their eating habits. Reading this book will enlighten you about the benefits of eating a good diet and the ways different food items help to boost and enhance the health of various organs of the body, thereby improving overall health. It also warns us against various hurdles that may come on the way to healthy eating, along with highlighting the negative impacts of adopting an unhealthy diet, which eventually has long-term effects on our health. The interesting part is that the book also has some fun-filled sections, that will make you aware of numerous myths that have bounded us for ages and a series of engaging facts that you may love to know and explore. On the whole, this book will make you the master of eating well and will surely change your lifestyle in a positive direction.

Lastly, I would like to thank all of you out there, who have spared your precious time to choose and read this book. I also appreciate the zeal within you, to take up the biggest challenge of life by standing against your cravings and opting for a healthy way of eating. I am glad to share with you all, that I am super excited to read your reviews for the book, as your feedbacks are really very precious to me and have the power to motivate me to write more entertaining books of your interest and choice. Before closing the book, let's descend deep into our minds and find the answers to the numerous mind-boggling questions that might be hovering within your head, like:

- Am I in good health?

- Do I have good eating habits?

- What should I eat to become fit and healthy?

- Do I follow a good diet plan?

- Which diet plan will be the best for me?

- Do I take sufficient calories?

- Is my diet supporting me to have a healthier me?

So, what are you all waiting for? The greatest opportunity is right before you, you just need to grab the book and get started with the beautiful journey of eating well and adopting a healthier lifestyle.

References

Alexander, H. (2020, July). *5 barriers to diet change and how to overcome them.* MD Anderson Cancer Center. https://www.mdanderson.org/publications/focused-on-health/5-barriers-to-diet-cange-and-how-to-overcome-them.h28-1593780.html

Arnarson, A. (2021, October 20). *Milk 101.* Healthline. https://www.healthline.com/nutrition/milk

Better Health Channel. (2012). *Cereals and wholegrain foods.* Better Health. https://www.betterhealth.vic.gov.au/health/HealthyLiving/cereals-and-wholegrain-foods

Bhuyan, N. (2022, May 18). *30 healthy eating quotes that will inspire workplace wellness.* Vantage Fit. https://www.vantagefit.io/blog/healthy-eating-quotes/

Biswas, C. (2014, March 21). *20 best healthy food quotes to inspire you.* Style Craze. https://www.stylecraze.com/articles/slogans-on-healthy-food/

Biswas, C. (2023, February 16). *16 positive effects of healthy eating on your life.* Style Craze. https://www.stylecraze.com/articles/positive-effects-of-healthy-eating-on-your-life/

Bjarnadottir, A. (2015). *Olives 101: Nutrition facts and health benefits.* Healthline. https://www.healthline.com/nutrition/foods/olives

Bjarnadottir, A. (2018, October 3). *The 5 best calorie counter websites and apps.* Healthline. https://www.healthline.com/nutrition/5-best-calorie-counters

Bulatseskul, G. (2017, January 5). *Nutrition and productivity: How foods can affect your performance.* Healthy Blog. https://foodtolive.com/healthy-blog/nutrition-productivity-foods-can-affect-performance/#:~:text=Such%20a%20diet%20can%20lead

Byju's. (n.d.). *Food sources- Food from plants, food from animals.* BYJUS. https://byjus.com/biology/food-sources-animal-plant-products/

Case, H. (n.d.). *Disadvantages of an unhealthy diet.* Live Strong. https://www.livestrong.com/article/194483-disadvantages-of-an-unhealthy-diet/

Creative World School. (2013, November 19). *Did you know: Healthy food facts.* Creative World School. https://creativeworldschool.com/did-you-know-healthy-food-facts/

Crichton-Stuart, C. (2020, December 10). *The top 10 benefits of eating healthy.* Medical News Today. https://www.medicalnewstoday.com/articles/322268

Deepika. (2022, March 30). *Types of diet plan: 7 different types of diet for weight loss.* Possible. https://possible.in/different-types-of-diets-for-weight-loss.html

Devje, S. (2019, September 25). *Meat: Good or bad?* Healthline Media. https://www.healthline.com/nutrition/meat-good-or-bad#cancer

Editorial Contributors, W. (2022, November 8). *Sleep-related eating disorders.* WebMD. https://www.webmd.com/sleep-disorders/sleep-related-eating-disorders

Elizabeth, E. (2022, August 30). *8 types of seafood you can eat.* Restaurant Clicks. https://restaurantclicks.com/types-of-seafood/

Elliott, B. (2017, August 9). *19 water-rich foods that help you stay hydrated.* Healthline. https://www.healthline.com/nutrition/19-hydrating-foods#TOC_TITLE_HDR_21

Food Standards Scotland. (2019, October 11). *The five main food groups - Healthy eating.* Food Standards Scotland. https://www.foodstandards.gov.scot/consumers/healthy-eating/nutrition/the-five-food-groups

Gemma. (2019, July 17). *20 fun facts about healthy eating.* Caribbean Green Living. https://www.caribbeangreenliving.com/20-fun-facts-about-healthy-eating/

Gunnars, K. (2018, March 27). *Top 10 nutrition facts that everyone agrees on.* Healthline. https://www.healthline.com/nutrition/top-10-nutrition-facts#TOC_TITLE_HDR_5

Gunnars, K. (2019, December 12). *Are vegetable and seed oils bad for your health?* Healthline. https://www.healthline.com/nutrition/are-vegetable-and-seed-oils-bad#:~:text=They%20are%20often%20labeled%20%E2%80%9Cheart

Harrington, R. (2023, January 3). *17 scientific facts to motivate you to eat healthier, even when you don't want to.* Business Insider. https://www.businessinsider.in/science/news/17-scientific-facts-to-motivate-you-to-eat-healthier-even-when-you-donapost-want-to/slidelist/96718342.cms

Harris, K. (2017, October 16). *18 quotes on food and health to make you think.* Treehugger. https://www.treehugger.com/quotes-on-food-and-health-that-will-make-you-think-4868766

Head, A. (2019, April 18). *23 healthy food habits that these celebrities credit feeling good to.* Women's Health. https://www.womenshealthmag.com/uk/food/healthy-eating/g27164610/celebrity-health-habits/

HealthKart. (2022, April 26). *Types of diet plans you should know about.* HealthKart. https://www.healthkart.com/connect/types-of-diet-plans-which-one-would-you-choose/

Hopkins, J. (2021, August 8). *ABCs of eating smart for a healthy heart.* Hopkins Medicine. https://www.hopkinsmedicine.org/health/wellness-and-prevention/abcs-of-eating-smart-for-a-healthy-heart

Horowitz, J. (2022, May 21). *Chloe Burrows in bathing suit says "My vibe right now."* Celebwell. https://celebwell.com/news-chloe-burrows-in-bathing-suit-says-my-vibe-right-now/

Hussein, J. (2018, July 26). *20 reasons you should be eating more fish.* Eat This Not That; Eat This Not That. https://www.eatthis.com/health-benefits-of-fish/

Jacob, D. (2021, November 10). *What are 10 benefits of eating vegetables?* MedicineNet. https://www.medicinenet.com/what_are_10_benefits_of_eating_vegetables/article.htm

Jamie. (2022, May 19). *23 different types of seafood with several benefits 2022.* Lacademie. https://www.lacademie.com/types-of-seafood/

Jennings, K.-A. (2023, February 27). *11 healthy-eating myths that just aren't true.* Food Network. https://www.foodnetwork.com/healthy/packages/healthy-every-week/healthy-tips/11-healthy-eating-myths-that-just-arent-true

Junejo, A. (2020, July 10). *Eat to live, live to eat.* Medium. https://aajunejo.medium.com/eat-to-live-live-to-eat-5045476d7dbc

Jyoti, A. (2021, March 22). *What are the main components of food.* Science Query. https://sciencequery.com/what-are-the-main-components-of-food/

Kataria, S. (2021, December 24). *40 Healthy eating quotes that motivate you to eat healthy.* Morning Lazziness. https://www.morninglazziness.com/quotes/healthy-eating-quotes/

Khanna, R. (2022a, May 7). *What is Tom Cruise's diet and workout routine that keeps him in great shape even after 50?* Sportskeeda. https://www.sportskeeda.com/health-and-fitness/what-tom-cruise-s-diet-workout-routine-keeps-great-shape-even-50

Khanna, R. (2022b, August 8). *Kate Hudson's diet and intense workout routine.* Sportskeeda. https://www.sportskeeda.com/health-and-fitness/kate-hudson-s-workout-diet-routine#:~:text=She%20avoids%20dairy%20and%20acidic

Kidadl Team. (2022, January 14). *Interesting and healthy food facts that we all should know.* Kidadl. https://kidadl.com/facts/interesting-and-healthy-food-facts-that-we-all-should-know

Knott, L. (2016, January 7). *Healthy eating.* Patient Info. https://patient.info/healthy-living/healthy-eating

Kubala, J. (2018, March 18). *5 proven health benefits of milk.* Healthline. https://www.healthline.com/nutrition/milk-benefits

Kubala, J. (2019, December 1). *23 ways to stop overeating.* Healthline. https://www.healthline.com/nutrition/how-to-stop-overeating#TOC_TITLE_HDR_2

Kubala, J. (2021, June 24). *Healthy eating 101: Nutrients, macros, tips, and more.* Healthline. https://www.healthline.com/nutrition/how-to-eat-healthy-guide

Leech, J. (2017, June 3). *10 delicious herbs and spices with powerful health benefits.* Healthline. https://www.healthline.com/nutrition/10-healthy-herbs-and-spices

Leech, J. (2019). *11 evidence-based health benefits of eating fish.* Healthline. https://www.healthline.com/nutrition/11-health-benefits-of-fish

Lehman, S. (2019). *Using the Harris-Benedict formula for calculating daily calorie intake.* Verywell Fit. https://www.verywellfit.com/how-many-calories-do-i-need-each-day-2506873

McClees, H. (2014, December 23). *Here's why non-dairy milk is a health choice, not health hype.* One Green Planet. https://www.onegreenplanet.org/natural-health/heres-why-non-dairy-milk-is-a-health-choice-not-health-hype/

McQueen, J. (2022, August 15). *Health benefits of legumes.* WebMD. https://www.webmd.com/food-recipes/health-benefits-legumes

Migala, J. (2018, August 29). *The importance of healthy eating habits.* EverydayHealth.com. https://www.everydayhealth.com/diet-nutrition/importance-healthy-eating-habits/

Mikstas, C. (2021, April 21). Slideshow: Health benefits of coffee and tea. WebMD. https://www.webmd.com/food-recipes/ss/slideshow-coffee-tea-benefits

Natale, N. (2022, February 10). *Watch Jennifer Aniston share the exercises that have her feeling her strongest at 52 in new IG video.* Prevention.https://www.prevention.com/life/a39028290/jennifer-aniston-at-home-workout-routine-instagram-video/

NDTV Food. (2018, February 23). *7 food facts you need to know to stay healthy.* NDTV Food. https://food.ndtv.com/food-drinks/7-food-facts-you-need-to-know-to-stay-healthy-1453724

NHS inform. (2020, April 30). *Health benefits of eating well.* NHS Inform. https://www.nhsinform.scot/healthy-living/food-and-nutrition/eating-well/health-benefits-of-eating-well

Pagán, C. N. (2022, March 3). *Diabetes and fruit*. WebMD. https://www.webmd.com/diabetes/fruit-diabetes#:~:text=a%20healthy%20weight.-

Parmar, R. (2022, March 1). *Top 11 health benefits of eating well*. PharmEasy Blog. https://pharmeasy.in/blog/top-9-health-benefits-of-eating-well/

Pathak, N. (2019, July 18). *Constituents of food and its functions*. James Lind Institute. https://www.jliedu.com/blog/constituents-food-functions/

Petre, A. (2022, April 11). *Learn about 6 common types of eating disorders and their symptoms*. Healthline. https://www.healthline.com/nutrition/common-eating-disorders#-6.-Avoidant/restrictive-food-intake-disorder

Pink, A., Wilkinson, L., Price, M., & Embling, R. (2020, November 9). *Food variety is important for our health — but the definition of a "balanced diet" is often murky*. The Conversation. https://theconversation.com/food-variety-is-important-for-our-health-but-the-definition-of-a-balanced-diet-is-often-murky-149126

Raman, R. (2019, August 5). *The 8 best diet plans — Sustainability, weight loss, and more*. Healthline Media. https://www.healthline.com/nutrition/best-diet-plans

Seeber, B. (2016, August 25). *7 ways to reduce salt intake and lower your blood pressure*. EverydayHealth. https://www.everydayhealth.com/columns/white-seeber-grogan-the-remedy-chicks/ways-to-reduce-salt-intake-every-day/

Spritzler, F. (2022, November 9). *Can apple cider vinegar help you lose weight?* Healthline. https://www.healthline.com/nutrition/apple-cider-vinegar-weight-loss

Staff, H. (2022, May 9). Health topics A-Z. PeaceHealth. https://www.peacehealth.org/medical-topics/id/nutri

Stein, N. (2018, December 17). *Disadvantages in poor nutrition.* Healthy Eating | SF Gate. https://healthyeating.sfgate.com/disadvantages-poor-nutrition-10928.html

Stiefvater, S. (2021, January 19). *9 healthy eating quotes to motivate you to make better choices.* PureWow. https://www.purewow.com/wellness/healthy-eating-quotes

Suni, E. (2020, November 6). *Nutrition and sleep: Diet's effect on sleep.* Sleep Foundation. https://www.sleepfoundation.org/nutrition

Suni, E. (2021, March 2). *The impact of an eating disorder on sleep.* Sleep Foundation. https://www.sleepfoundation.org/mental-health/eating-disorders-and-sleep

Tighe, M. (2013, February 21). *Healthy eating obstacles.* Trillium Natural Medicine. http://www.trilliumnatural.com/2013/02/healthy-eating-obstacles/

Times of India. (2021, October 21). *Boiled lemon water: Benefits of drinking it and ways to make it.* The Times of India. https://timesofindia.indiatimes.com/life-style/health-fitness/diet/boiled-lemon-water-benefits-of-drinking-it-and-ways-to-make-it/photostory/87162889.cms#:~:text=If%20you%20are%20one%20of

Unoreads. (2021, August 17). Components of food. Unoreads. https://www.unoreads.com/article/components-of-food

Urja. (2016, April 25). *How to create your own diet plan·* HealthKart. https://www.healthkart.com/connect/how-to-create-your-own-diet-plan/bid-4278

Vyas, A. (2019, March 25). *Importance of healthy eating habits in our life.* Radiance Hospitals. https://www.radiancehospitals.org/blog/healthy-eating-habits/

Waldbieser, J. (2020, April 20). *19 food facts that may change how you eat.* The Healthy. https://www.thehealthy.com/food/unbelievable-food-facts-that-will-change-how-you-eat/

Wartenberg, L. (2020, November 20). *Frozen yogurt vs. ice cream: Is one healthier?* Healthline. https://www.healthline.com/nutrition/frozen-yogurt-vs-ice-cream#benefits

West, H. (2016, June 7). *Counting calories 101: How to count calories to lose weight.* Healthline Media. https://www.healthline.com/nutrition/counting-calories-101

Whelan, C. (2017, October 14). *Fruit diet: Benefits, risks, and more.* Healthline. https://www.healthline.com/health/food-nutrition/fruit-diet#potential-benefits

Y, S. (2022, August 25). *Lucy Liu's healthy lifestyle tips for looking good and feeling great.* Sportskeeda. https://www.sportskeeda.com/health-and-fitness/lucy-liu-s-healthy-lifestyle-tips#:~:text=Lucy%20Liu

Zafar, S. (2022, September 9). *The benefits of plant-based oils.* Bio Energy Consult. https://www.bioenergyconsult.com/benefits-of-plant-based-oils/

Zambon, V. (2021, January 21). *Counting calories: What to know to lose or gain weight.* Medical News Today. https://www.medicalnewstoday.com/articles/counting-calories

Image References

Ayrton, A. (2021, January 20). *Woman showing apple and bitten doughnut [Online Image]*. Pexels. https://www.pexels.com/photo/woman-showing-apple-and-bitten-doughnut-6551415/

Doan, J. (2018, January 14). *Variety of food on wooden coaster [Online Image]*. Pexels. https://www.pexels.com/photo/variety-of-food-on-wooden-coaster-793759/

Gabor, A. (2018, September 15). *Assorted vegetables on brown wooden table [Online Image]*. Pexels. https://www.pexels.com/photo/assorted-vegetables-on-brown-wooden-table-1414651/

Grabowska, K. (2020, June 1). *Empty clipboard with fresh vegetables and herbs on table [Online Images]*. Pexels. https://www.pexels.com/photo/empty-clipboard-with-fresh-vegetables-and-herbs-on-table-4033636/

Jordan, J. J. (2021, August 21). *Yellow and red round fruit on brown and white weighing scale [Online Image]*. Pexels. https://www.pexels.com/photo/yellow-and-red-round-fruit-on-brown-and-white-weighing-scale-9241897/

Miroshnichenko, T. (2021, May 13). *A person carrying steel basket with assorted fruits and Vvgetables [Online Image]*. Pexels. https://www.pexels.com/photo/a-person-carrying-steel-basket-with-assorted-fruits-and-vegetables-7879964/

Pixabay. (2017, July 19). *Close-up of salad on table [Online Image]*. Pexels. https://www.pexels.com/photo/close-up-of-salad-on-table-326281/

RODNAE Productions. (2021, June 17). *Person holding gold wedding band [Online Image]*. Pexels. https://www.pexels.com/photo/food-wood-light-man-8370777/

Scramgnon, B. (2017, October 2). *Bowl of cereal with raisins [Online Image]*. Pexels. https://www.pexels.com/photo/bowl-of-cereal-with-raisins-596133/

Shekhovtcova, A. (2021, February 24). *Forks with fried potatoes with ketchup on yellow background [Online Image]*. Pexels. https://www.pexels.com/photo/forks-with-fried-potatoes-with-ketchup-on-yellow-background-6941028/

Shuraev, Y. (2021, July 21). *A woman making a meal plan [Online Image]*. Pexels. https://www.pexels.com/photo/a-woman-making-a-meal-plan-8844383/

Stone, S. (2022, June 15). *Glass of water beside slices of apple and record on calorie count on brown wooden table [Online Images]*. Pexels. https://www.pexels.com/photo/glass-of-water-beside-slices-of-apple-and-record-on-calorie-count-on-brown-wooden-table-12499374/

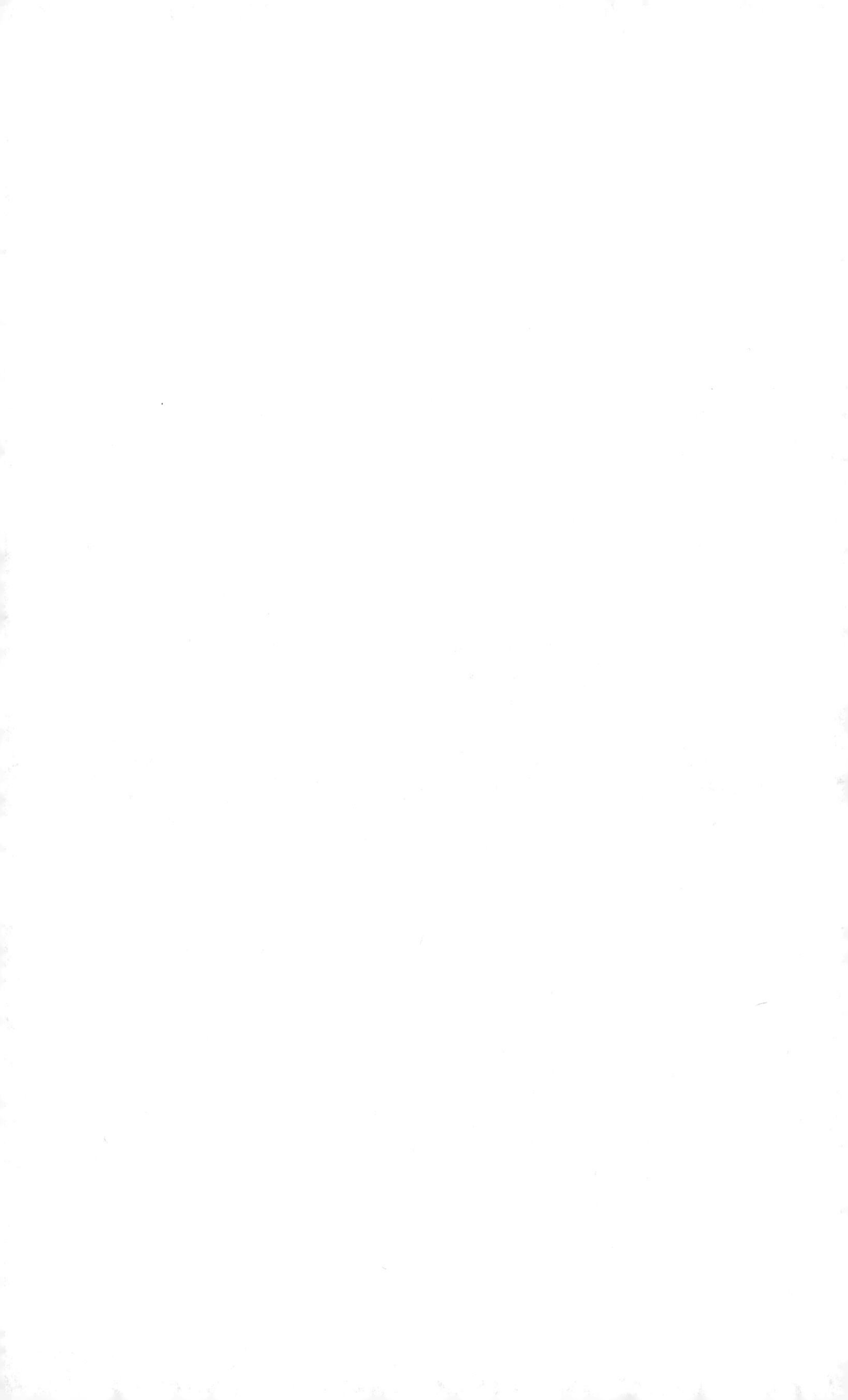

www.ingramcontent.com/pod-product-compliance
Lightning Source LLC
Chambersburg PA
CBHW070834250726
48662CB00003B/1224